30 Essential Yoga Poses

Also by Judith Lasater, Ph.D., P.T.

Relax and Renew:
Restful Yoga for Stressful Times
(Rodmell Press, 1995)

Living Your Yoga:
Finding the Spiritual
in Everyday Life
(Rodmell Press, 2000)

Judith Lasater, Ph.D., P.T.

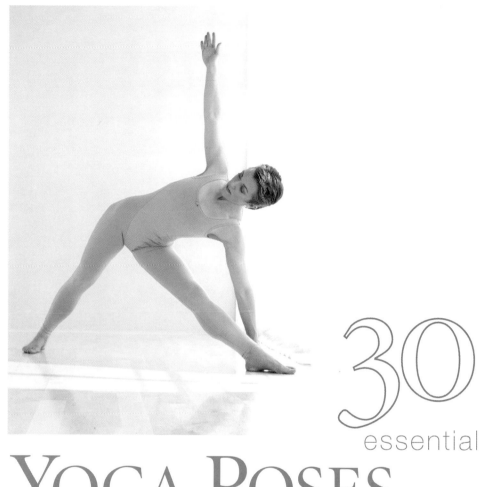

30 essential
YOGA POSES

FOR BEGINNING STUDENTS AND THEIR TEACHERS

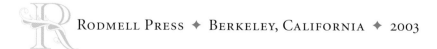
RODMELL PRESS ✦ BERKELEY, CALIFORNIA ✦ 2003

To my mother, Mildred Felix Miles Hanson, my first teacher

Library of Congress Cataloging-in-Publication Data

Lasater, Judith.
  30 essential yoga poses : for beginning students and their teachers /
Judith Lasater. — 1st ed.
    p. cm.
Includes bibliographical references and index.
  ISBN 1-930485-04-2 (pbk. : alk. paper)
  1. Yoga, Hātha. I. Title: Thirty essential yoga poses. II. Title.
  RA781.7.L367 2003
  613.7'046—dc21

                          2003013097

Printed in China
First Edition
ISBN 1-930485-04-2
10 09 08 07 06 05 04 03 1 2 3 4 5 6 7 8 9 10

Editor: Linda Cogozzo   Cover and Text Designer: Gopa & Ted2, Inc.
Copy Editor: Katherine L. Kaiser   Cover and Interior Photographer: David Martinez
Indexer: Ty Koontz   Author Photographer: Elizabeth Lasater
                                         Lithographer: Leo Paper Group

Text set in Minion

CONTENTS

Acknowledgments   vii

PART ONE: Beginning with an Ancient Tradition   1

About Yoga   2

About the Book   3

Go for the Joy   4

PART TWO: Being a Student, Being a Teacher   5

The Student Chooses the Teacher   6

Boundaries: Creating a Restorative Environment   6

Essential Guidelines for Students Attending a Yoga Class   8

Transitioning From Student to Teacher   9

Essential Guidelines for Teachers   9

From Colleague to Colleague   11

PART THREE: The Poses   13

1 Mountain Pose   15

2 Tree Pose   19

3 Extended Triangle Pose   25

4 Half-Moon Pose   31

5 Warrior I Pose   37

6 Warrior II Pose   43

7 Extended Side-Angle Stretch Pose   49

8 Side-Chest Stretch Pose   55

9 Wide-Leg Standing Forward Bend Pose   61

10 Downward-Facing Dog Pose   67

11 Standing Forward Bend Pose   73

12 Up-Plank Pose and Down-Plank Pose   79

13 Headstand Preparation Pose 85

14 Lunge Pose 91

15 Cobra Pose 97

16 Bow Pose 103

17 Bridge Pose 109

18 Upward-Facing Bow Pose 115

19 Elevated Legs-up-the-Wall Pose 121

20 Supported Shoulderstand Pose 127

21 Simple Seated-Twist Pose 133

22 Hero–Heroine Pose 139

23 Head-of-the-Knee Pose 145

24 Seated-Angle Pose 151

25 Bound-Angle Pose 157

26 Reclining Leg-Stretch Pose 163

27 Lying Twist Pose 169

28 Child's Pose 175

29 Basic Meditation Pose 179

30 Basic Relaxation Pose and
Essential Breathing Practices 185

PART FOUR: The Practice 195

The Sacred Circle 196

Sequencing and Why It Matters 196

Props and Why They Matter 197

Practical Tips for Practice 197

Four Practice Choices 198

Part Five: And More 237

Glossary 238

Resources 240

About the Model 242

About the Author 243

From the Publisher 244

Index 245

ACKNOWLEDGMENTS

THERE IS NO WAY TO THANK all the people who make the writing of a book possible. Nonetheless, I would like to try.

I thank my immediate and extended family for their constant encouragement. I extend special appreciation to my husband, Ike, for his expertise in communication and his willingness to share it with me. I thank my children—Miles, Kam, and Elizabeth—for their ability to help me repeatedly redefine practice throughout the years.

I acknowledge my very first yoga teachers, Sally and David Elsberry, who gave me the gift of my first yoga class and encouraged me to begin teaching so many years ago.

Without a doubt, my understanding of yoga would be significantly less without the practice and life of B. K. S. Iyengar, of Pune, India. I salute his dedication to the art of yoga, and am grateful for the knowledge and passion for practice that he has shared with me.

Namaste to my friends and colleagues Stephen Cope, John Friend, Lilias Folan, Elise Miller, and Richard Miller, for giving of themselves to this book and their heartfelt praise for this work.

My gratitude goes to the editorial and design team for their expertise and vision: editor Linda Cogozzo; Gopa and Veetam, the designers at Gopa & Ted2, Inc.; copy editor Katherine L. Kaiser; and indexer Ty Koontz.

I am especially thankful to the crew who made the photographs possible: yoga teacher Theresa Elliott, for her patient and enthusiastic modeling; photographer David Martinez, who created images that are not only beautiful, but also effective practice and teaching aids; Mark Dawson, for his technical expertise and good humor; France Dushane, for hair, makeup, and her gentle ways; studio manager Aneata Hagy, for her skillful organization behind the scenes; Lylia Baylin and Jeff Mason, caterers extraordinaire; and Shelly Martinez, for her uplifting presence.

My appreciation goes to those people and companies who generously gave us their products to photograph: Hollie Brinkman, Emily Dalton, and Eric Johnson at Hugger-Mugger Yoga Products; Marie Wright at Marie Wright Yoga Wear; and Whitney Winter at the Meco Corporation.

I am grateful to my publishers, Donald Moyer and Linda Cogozzo, at Rodmell Press, for their practical advice, which was of immeasurable help in shaping this book.

Finally, I thank my students, from whom I have learned the most about yoga, about teaching, and about myself.

PART ONE

BEGINNING WITH AN ANCIENT TRADITION

THIRTY ESSENTIAL YOGA POSES is designed to support your understanding of yoga through a well-rounded practice. I wrote the book for you, the student, even if you are at the most beginning level, as well as for your teachers. To study and teach yoga is to learn about yourself, especially about the abilities of your body and mind, as well as the challenges that they present to wholeness. Although the practice of yoga is a lifetime study, you can begin it simply and directly, a little at a time. When approached this way, learning about yourself is a discovery process that is fascinating, that is satisfying, and that will remain forever delightfully unfinished.

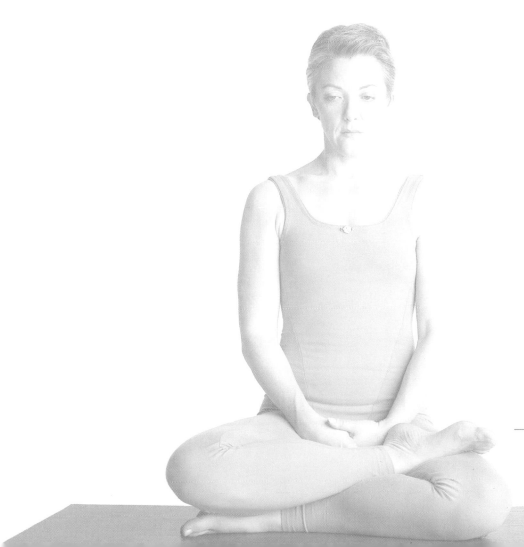

About Yoga

Classical yoga is a philosophical system that has its roots in ancient India. It remains vital today because yoga addresses the fundamental questions that we all face about health, awareness, and a life well lived. Although *yoga* is now a household word in the West, its philosophical background is not well known or understood here.

Yoga comes from Sanskrit, the scriptural language of ancient India. Its root is *yuj,* which means "to yoke" or "to unite." The Yoga Sutra of Patanjali, written in approximately 200 B.C.E., is generally accepted as the ultimate source book of classical yoga. In this revered text, Patanjali, who is thought to have been a physician, Sanskrit scholar, grammarian, and yogi, presents *astanga yoga,* or an "eight-limbed path" of practice.

The path begins with ten ethical precepts called *yamas* (restraints) and *niyamas* (observances). Called the first limb, the five yamas are *ahimsa* (nonharming), *satya* (truthfulness), *asteya* (nonstealing), *bramacharya* (clarity about sexual activity), and *aparighha* (nongreed). Georg Feuerstein, author of the *Encyclopedic Dictionary of Yoga,* says that the yamas "make up '*maha-vrata*' (the great vow) of the *yogin* [and *yogini*] and are to be practiced on all levels, irrespective of time, place, and circumstance."[1] The niyamas, which comprise the second limb, are *shauca* (purity), *samtosha* (contentment), *tapas* (discipline), *svadhyaya* (self-study), and *ishvara pranidhana* (surrender to God).

The third and fourth limbs, respectively, are asana (posture) and pranayama (breath control). My study of asana and pranayama has been influenced by the work of B. K. S. Iyengar, author of the classic text *Light on Yoga* and numerous other books. In 1974 and 1976, I studied with him at various venues in the United States. In addition, I have traveled three times to the Ramamani Iyengar Memorial Yoga Institute, in Pune, India, to study with him and his daughter, Geeta Iyengar. I am grateful to Mr. Iyengar and to Geeta Iyengar for their teaching, which inspires my own.

The fifth limb is *pratyahara* (the conscious withdrawal from the agitation of the senses). The sixth limb is *dharana* (concentration), the seventh limb is *dhyana* (meditation), and the eighth limb is *samadhi* (oneness). Taken together, the eight limbs help to develop self-awareness.

The practice of asana is the most easily recognized limb of yoga in the West. But, as can be seen from this brief introduction, asana is only a part of the whole picture of yoga practice. Although it is not my intention to offer instruction in all the limbs of Patanjali's yoga, I have woven their principles into the text. For example, do you practice *aparighha* (nongreed) when you covet another student's pose, wishing that you could do an advanced one as well?

It is my belief that no limb of yoga can be separated from the whole tree of its existence. Just as humans are complex beings who exist on a multiplicity of levels, yoga, if it is to serve such beings, must be studied on its many levels as well. References for continued study are listed in "Resources," which can be found in Part Five, "And More."

---

1. Georg Feuerstein, *Encyclopedic Dictionary of Yoga* (New York: Paragon House, 1990), 410.

ABOUT THE BOOK

I have organized *30 Essential Yoga Poses* in a way that I hope will encourage and simplify your practice. Part One, "Beginning with an Ancient Tradition," is a general overview of the philosophical foundation of yoga and why it is relevant today.

Part Two, "Being a Student, Being a Teacher," focuses on the student–teacher relationship. In earlier times, the yoga teacher worked with his or her student on a one-to-one basis. Today, most of yoga is taught in a class setting. Regardless of the forum, the relationship between student and teacher is essential to yoga. The teacher, who has presumably traversed the landscape, leads the student on his or her journey over the same terrain. And the relationship is a mutual one: the teacher learns from the student along the way.

It is my deep wish to educate students and teachers alike about the learning potential within this relationship. Not only do I give suggestions to help students learn more effectively should they choose to attend yoga classes, but I also offer guidelines to help teachers do their jobs with more awareness, knowledge, and compassion.

The thirty essential yoga poses are introduced in Part Three, "The Poses." I begin my discussion of each pose with my reflections. Then I describe how to sequence the pose with other poses; I follow this with the benefits and cautions. Next come nuts and bolts guidelines in what I call "The Essential Pose": what props are necessary; how to set up for the pose; the experience of the pose itself; and how to come out of the pose. I detail variations for each pose. As such, there are actually ninety-six poses presented in *30 Essential Yoga Poses*.

Part Three also includes specific information for teachers in "Primary Focus" and "Primary Adjustment." The former points out what to keep in mind when teaching the pose. The latter discusses what not to overlook when you help the student experience a more comfortable and enriched pose. Even if you do not teach yoga, I invite you to consult the sections for teachers, where you will find helpful suggestions for your personal practice.

Part Four, "The Practice," puts the poses together into coherent sequences. To open you to the possibilities that yoga philosophy offers, I include intentions for each practice session, which I call "Mantra for Daily Practice." The mantras are short, poignant phrases or sentences intended to help you gather your thoughts and declare an intention for your practice that day. In addition, I state the purpose of each sequence, and offer encouragement to my colleagues in "A Word to Teachers."

The first sequence is called "Busy Days Practice," for when there doesn't seem to be any time at all for yoga. The next approach is called "Day-of-the-Week Practice," which divides the thirty essential poses into seven daily practices. This easy-to-follow guide covers all the poses, either the essential pose or a variation, in a week.

The third approach is called "Theme Practice." For example, you can choose to concentrate on your lower back, or on flexibility for your hamstrings, or on your upper back and shoulders. Alternatively, you can choose to spend a practice session working on improving your balance, increasing your overall strength, reducing your fatigue, or creating relaxation. I encourage teachers to use these sequences in planning classes. Finally, the last section of Part Four is "The 30 Essential Yoga Poses Practice," and is intended for days when you have the time and inclination to devote yourself to an in-depth practice.

Once you decide on which practice approach you want to follow on any specific day, you will find an illustrated list of poses to accomplish your goals. If needed, you can refer back to Part Three, where detailed instructions are given for each of those poses.

Finally, Part Five, "And More," presents a glossary of anatomical terms and resources.

Go for the Joy

In my early twenties, I chose to take my first yoga class to improve my health. Yoga stuck with me: I stuck with yoga. My personal study of yoga quickly became a passion that manifested itself in my own regular daily practice and evolved to include teaching others. Since 1971, I have enjoyed sharing yoga practice in classes and workshops worldwide.

In *30 Essential Yoga Poses,* I try to share with you the joy I get from practicing and teaching yoga. More important, I hope that the book inspires you to find your own joy, and to create and sustain your own personal home practice. I also hope that this book offers information and stimulation to my fellow yoga teachers, who continuously strive to refine their skills in the important art of teaching. My warmest and best wishes as you continue your own discovery of the ancient–and yet eternally new–study, practice, and teaching of yoga.

PART TWO

BEING A STUDENT, BEING A TEACHER

Your impetus to practice yoga may be physical, such as a desire to increase your flexibility or to reduce the toll of stress on your body. Or you may want to experience equanimity or to gain spiritual insight. Or perhaps the yoga class was the only class with any openings at your local community center. Whatever your reason, yoga is an adventure of self-discovery.

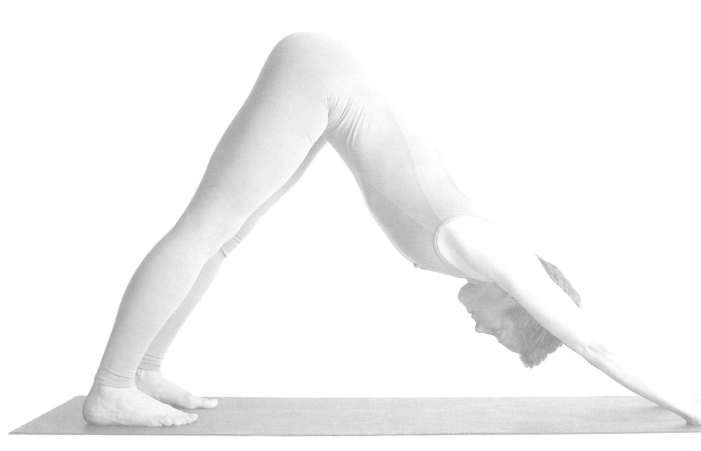

Some students prefer to explore yoga on their own, studying from books and practicing at home. But most likely you study yoga with a teacher, and you use books and other resources to reinforce your practice in between classes. An ongoing relationship with a teacher can be a valuable tool that facilitates self-awareness. This relationship is powerful: it is useful to examine it in depth. This part of the book does just that.

Although some information is for students and some is for teachers, I encourage all readers to examine this part thoroughly. If you are a student, you may find that understanding the viewpoint of your teacher and his or her challenges helps you to become a more focused student. If you are a teacher, remembering the concerns of your students will undoubtedly stimulate the compassion necessary to teach.

The Student Chooses the Teacher

You may be so conditioned by years of schooling that you no longer question what it means to be a student. The student–teacher relationship in yoga is different from the relationships that you had with your teachers in school. The primary difference is that you as the yoga student have much more responsibility than you had in school.

To be a yoga student is to take charge of your own practice, your own growth, and your own life in ways that you may never have done before. To be a yoga student is to remain conscious of the *process* of learning, not just the *content* of what you are learning. You may find it interesting and enlightening to observe how you react to difficult poses as well as easy ones. What comes up for you in the learning process? Do you expect to learn quickly and become frustrated when you do not? If you remain aware of the process of learning, then the lessons of the poses can be taken from the experiences that you have on the mat and applied to the experiences of living your life, minute by minute and even thought by thought.

It is you, the student, who chooses your teacher. Paradoxically, the primary relationship that you have in yoga practice is with yourself. As you practice the poses, you begin to notice how you speak to yourself, what you demand of yourself, and how you judge yourself. When something is difficult, do you admonish yourself or do you encourage yourself? Do you approach a challenge good-naturedly or do you mutter about your shortcomings under your breath?

The same is true for the teacher. Each teacher experiences a relationship with herself as she practices. The quality of this relationship with the self will be expressed during the act of teaching a class. *A teacher cannot teach any differently from how she practices.* Inevitably, the internal relationship a teacher has with her personal practice is revealed through her attitude, actions, and language in class. So check out the teacher. Is your need for respect met when she speaks to you or adjusts you in a pose? Does your teacher sometimes cross a verbal or physical boundary which you would prefer be maintained? These observations can lead you to find a class that meets your needs for safety and respect.

Boundaries: Creating a Restorative Environment

It is the job of the yoga teacher to create and maintain a healthful environment in which he or she can teach and the student can learn. A vital component of such an environment is boundaries. Rooted in yoga's ethical precepts, the *yamas* and *niyamas,* which I discuss in Part One, "Beginning with an Ancient Tradition," these boundaries are not just a dry list of prohibitions and prescriptions, but point toward what is best for both teacher and student. *The most important aspect of the student–teacher relationship is the clarity with which these boundaries are created and maintained.* This may sound like a strong statement: it is intended to be one. From this clarity comes trust, and from trust comes relaxation and growth.

Jungian psychoanalyst Jean Shinoda Bolen, M.D., author of *Goddesses in Everywoman: A New Psychology of Women,* describes what she calls the "sacred circle." Here is my understanding of Dr. Bolen's idea.[1] When a teacher enters the teaching situation, especially when this situation is concerned with spiritual or personal evolution, the teacher's first responsibility is to create a sacred circle of safety and awareness, so that the student can feel completely safe in exploring all aspects of himself, in his own way, and in his own time.

I find this concept so compelling that I include techniques for creating it even when practicing alone at home. You will find these techniques in Part Four, "The Practice." Simply put, whether you are a student or a teacher, the more you work with creating and maintaining your own boundaries, the better you will understand a healthful student–teacher relationship.

Just by walking in the door of a classroom, the student has entered the sacred circle of the student–teacher relationship. However, this sacred circle exists not only in the classroom but also in the wider relationship between the student and the teacher. It is the responsibility of the teacher to acknowledge and guard the safety of the student. This safety extends to the physical, mental, emotional, psychological, sexual, financial, and spiritual realms. In practical terms, it means that a teacher does not date or have sex with his or her students, does not become enmeshed in their private or financial lives, and does not take on the role of a psychotherapist.

The key to understanding this student–teacher boundary is simple: *The teacher is to consider all of his or her actions against a backdrop of the student's welfare.* Whatever action the teacher takes, whether it be to physically adjust the student in a pose, to speak with another teacher about a teaching dilemma, or to consider going out for tea with a student after class, this action must be weighed with the student's best interest in mind.

It is inappropriate for the teacher to act from self-interest in the student–teacher relationship. Any attempt by the teacher to use the student–teacher relationship for his or her own ends violates the boundary between student and teacher, an act that can have important and often negative effects for the student. You need only to examine the history of fallen gurus to be reminded of how much trust the student puts into the student–teacher relationship, and how important it is for the teacher to respect that trust.

The student has responsibility as well. It behooves the student to remain an active, discriminating member of the student–teacher dyad. Although the teacher has the professional responsibility to respect and protect the student, the student has the responsibility to take care of himself or herself. See "Essential Guidelines for Students Attending a Yoga Class," which follows. When both teacher and student act from a place of respect—respect for the self and respect for the other—the process of learning and self-discovery is easier and more fulfilling.

Finally and most important, things go better when the yoga teacher remains professional, that is, when the teacher understands his or her role: a guide who is friendly but not necessarily a friend and a supporter who remains apart from, but not separate from, the personal life of his or her student.

---

1. Jean Shinoda Bolen, M.D., personal conversation with the author, 1990.

ESSENTIAL GUIDELINES
FOR STUDENTS ATTENDING A YOGA CLASS

If you choose to practice yoga in a class setting, here are some guidelines to consider. As you will discover, many of them are ways to work with boundaries. Practical guidelines—when to eat, why remove your watch, what to wear, and others—can be found in Part Four, "The Practice."

PREPARE WITH CARE. Getting ready for class can be a ritual that helps you get into the right frame of mind for concentrating on your practice. If possible, shower before you come to class and wear clean practice clothes. Make sure that these clothes are comfortable and modest, and wear underwear. Remember that you might be turning upside down, and so a low-cut top (if you are a woman) or wide-legged shorts (if you are a man) may reveal more than you would be comfortable with showing. If you need to change clothing when you get to class, do it in a designated area, such as the bathroom.

BE ON TIME. Arrive on time for class, and arrange your schedule so that you do not have to leave early. Doing this is a manifestation of your respect for yourself, your teacher, your fellow students, and the ancient tradition of yoga.

MOTIVATION. Be clear about your motivation for practice, and renew your commitment to practice on an ongoing basis. You can do this by developing and maintaining a daily home practice, and by silently stating your practice intention as you step onto the mat. Before you panic, wondering how you will fit yoga practice into an already crowded day, consider that you can commit to little as five minutes a day. The highest form of discipline is consistency: powerful transformation can come from regularity. I suggest ways to practice and practice intentions in Part Four, "The Practice."

WHAT A YOGA TEACHER IS NOT. Keep in mind that your yoga teacher is someone who teaches poses, breathing exercises, and meditation. He or she is not your doctor or psychotherapist. Think of your teacher as one of your health care advisers. You can take him or her into your confidence about your physical and mental state, but do not project onto your teacher more healing ability than is warranted.

TRUST YOURSELF. Listen to your body and remember that you are in charge. Although your teacher is your respected guide, you are the ultimate authority on what is right for you at every moment of your life. If a pose seems to be too much for you right now, then you can practice part of it, or modify it with props, or let it go for today and try it at another time.

HONOR YOURSELF. Accept the teacher's physical adjustments and verbal instructions that are appropriate for you. If you are unhappy with either one (or with anything else about the class), then speak to your teacher after class, stating your preferences with firmness and clarity. No matter how wonderful an adjustment is, if you are not ready for it, then it is not appropriate.

COMMUNICATION. Speak with your teacher if the state of your health has changed significantly. It is best to discuss your health with your teacher privately, because class is a group experience, and the teacher must pay attention to the concerns of all class members.

HUMOR. Keeping a sense of humor about yourself, your practice, and your class will help not only you, but also your teacher and the others who practice with you.

TRANSITIONING FROM STUDENT TO TEACHER

Every teacher begins as a student. After taking classes for some time, you may feel drawn toward becoming a teacher. The first requirement for being a teacher is to be a consistent practitioner. If you have not yet established a daily home practice, then do that first before you begin to study to become a teacher.

If you are sure that you want to proceed, then talk to your teacher outside of class. Ask him or her to honestly evaluate your potential as a teacher. You may want to apprentice with your teacher or another teacher whom your teacher recommends. Helping a teacher to teach a class will give you a taste of what teaching is like.

If apprenticing whets your appetite, then ask your teacher what training programs he or she recommends. Spend some time checking out the programs. There is no required legal accreditation of yoga teachers in the United States. Consequently, the length of training programs ranges from a weekend to three years.

To find a teacher training program that is right for you, talk to several students currently in that program, as well as to that program's graduates. Ask them about the quality of the training and how they are using it in their lives, both professionally and personally. Pick the program that resonates with you, and then study with a whole heart. Most important, remember that even when you become a teacher you will always remain a student of yoga.

ESSENTIAL GUIDELINES FOR TEACHERS

Teaching yoga can be challenging and rewarding. It is often just plain fun as well. Yoga teachers usually have the chance to create their own schedule. Yoga teachers are paid to interact with people in ways that are about becoming healthier on all levels. And we get to do all this while barefoot! Many consider this to be the perfect job.

No matter how many classes you have taught, each one is new and offers a unique experience. Even if the students facing you have studied with you for decades, this class, this pose, and this moment are absolutely new. Following are some reminders to help you create a restorative environment.

THE DIVINE. Your student is a manifestation of the Divine. Treat him or her with the respect that you would wish for yourself.

A TWO-WAY STREET. Practice what you teach: teach what you practice. Your students have chosen *you* to teach them. Trust what you have experienced in your practice and let it show.

DAILY PRACTICE. Having a consistent daily practice is the foundation necessary to teaching well. When you practice every day, not only do you renew yourself for your next class, but you also model to your students the power and importance of a daily personal practice.

MOTIVATION. Understand your motivation to teach. When you check in with yourself, I hope that you discover that your primary motivation is to serve your students in love and compassion. Renew this commitment on a regular basis. One way that I do this is by repeating my life goal to myself before every class: I teach to facilitate humankind's reconnection with the Sacred. I use this life goal to guide me when I am not sure of what course to take, what asana to teach, or what to say to an upset student. I try to act in a way that is consistent with my goal, because I feel that if we all reconnect with the Sacred, as we perceive the Sacred to be, then together we can solve all the problems of the world. When I focus on this life goal, I find it easier to approach my teaching as service, and I remain focused on the students' learning instead of my performance as a teacher.

TEACH WHAT YOU KNOW. Understand that the job of a yoga teacher to teach yoga. Know when you don't know, and know when it is time to refer your student to a health care professional. Remember that although yoga can be a great boon to health, it is not a cure-all.

FEEDBACK. Do not isolate yourself. Seek out other teachers at classes, at conferences, at trainings, and online. It is amazing how much support you can gain from such relationships. Many teachers find it helpful to attend a monthly forum in which teachers take turns teaching a class and giving each other feedback and support when requested. If no such forum exists, consider creating one.

WHAT TO WEAR. Dress professionally. A yoga teacher wears form-fitting exercise clothes, so that students can see the asana when he or she demonstrates them. Pay attention to the importance of clear boundaries when making your wardrobe selection. For example, do not reveal the upper third of your thigh. If you are a woman, do not wear a low-cut top that reveals your breasts. If you are a man, wear a T-shirt.

PREPARATION. Come to class prepared to teach. Some teachers like to plan each pose that they are going to teach: others are more spontaneous. Whatever your style (and either is effective), spend a few quiet minutes before you teach reconnecting with your intention for the upcoming class. This intention can be something as simple as to remember to breathe between instructions or to remember to interact with that student in the back row whom you always seem to ignore.

BE ON TIME. Begin and end your class on time. Remember that students have lives outside of your class. They have babysitters and children who are waiting, or appointments with their accountants, or jobs to go to after class. Be there on time to show your dedication to teaching; end on time to show your respect for your students.

MAY I TOUCH YOU? Create safety in making adjustments. I ask the question, May I touch you?, and wait for the student to answer me *each* time with *each* student in *each* class, regardless of how many years that student may have taken my classes. I do this for three reasons. First, it lets the student know that I will not touch her without permission. This allows the student to relax when I am behind her or when she is lying down relaxing with her eyes closed.

Second, my asking telegraphs to other students in the class that they are in a safe environment: I will not trespass on their own personal space. Finally, asking permission to touch each time reminds *me* as the teacher that I am about to enter the sacred space of someone else. Asking helps me remember to slow down and enter that space with compassion and clear intention.

WORDS. Choose your words carefully. They can inspire, cajole, intimidate, or support. They can be as potent as any physical adjustment, and may echo in the ears of your student long after he or she leaves class.

USE HUMOR. Laughter releases tension from the diaphragm, lowers blood pressure, improves immune function, and releases endorphins. The practice of yoga is too important to be serious.

BE YOURSELF. Remember that you are not only teaching poses, breathing practices, and meditation techniques: you are also sharing skills to help your students live with courage and someday die with grace. Do not worry that you may not know enough. No one does. Be yourself.

FROM COLLEAGUE TO COLLEAGUE

The role of teacher is a multilayered one. Although I do not always have the answers to the following questions, I have found it helpful to consider them. Just asking myself these questions helps me to look more deeply at myself.

MOTIVATION. Do you need to be in absolute control of the class, or do you allow for a little give and take, for questions, and for the occasional appropriate joke from a student? Are you seeking approval from your students? How do you respond when asked a difficult question, or a question to which you do not know the answer? Periodically, review your motivation for teaching. Being flexible is good for your hamstrings—and good for your life. Creating a relaxed and supportive environment in your classes will model for your students a way of being in the world that is healthy for them as well as you.

CRITICIZING OTHER TEACHERS. I feel uncomfortable when I hear yoga teachers publicly criticize other teachers, systems, or spiritual traditions. How do you handle questions from students that would allow you or your system to seem superior to another teacher or system? Do you take the bait or tactfully say, "I don't know why teacher X or system Y teaches the pose that way, but let me explain why I teach it the way I do." Shifting the emphasis *from* what is wrong with them *to* this is what I would like you to do is not only more tactful and professional, but also a great way to keep the class from getting bogged down in criticism and negativity.

TALKING ABOUT OTHER STUDENTS. In addition to avoiding talking about other teachers in class, avoid talking about one of your students with another one of your students outside of class. If you talk about another student, then you create mistrust: you appear to disrespect the first student, and you make the second student uncomfortable. If you do discuss your students with one another, have you examined your motivation for doing so?

SOCIALIZING WITH STUDENTS. Have you consciously chosen your boundaries? Do you socialize with your students? Some teachers living in small communities tell me that if they didn't socialize with their students, then they would have no social life, because their students are the only ones with similar interests. More important than whether you socialize with your students is the clarity with which you choose your boundaries. Do you keep the welfare of the student foremost in your mind, or are you more interested in what you can gain from the relationship? Who has more to lose if the relationship falls apart?

BURNOUT. Are you dragging yourself to class to teach? Are you unable to find the time to practice as much as you would like? Are you tired all the time? Maybe you are burned out. Teaching yoga is physically and emotionally demanding. Allowing adequate time between classes is critical. One common pattern is to teach in the evening and then again first thing the next morning. Many teachers find this combination especially draining. Can you create a schedule that is sustainable?

I strongly suggest that all yoga teachers take at least three weeks off each year from teaching. If you let your students know of your plans well in advance, then they can plan their vacations, too, after which you can all return refreshed and ready to study together again.

FURTHER STUDY. In addition to taking time off, take time to pursue further study for yourself so that you can reconnect with the experience of being a student. That study might be taking a yoga seminar, or it might mean taking a class in something that seems completely unrelated. The key is to choose something that will renew your spirit. You can give only from a full cup: offering the gift of yoga in the spirit of that fullness is the core of great teaching.

The best teachers are those who are the best students. And in a way, we are all teachers because we always have at least ourselves as students. I hope that this discussion about the interplay of teaching and studying yoga will enrich your understanding of learning and embolden your teaching.

PART THREE

THE POSES

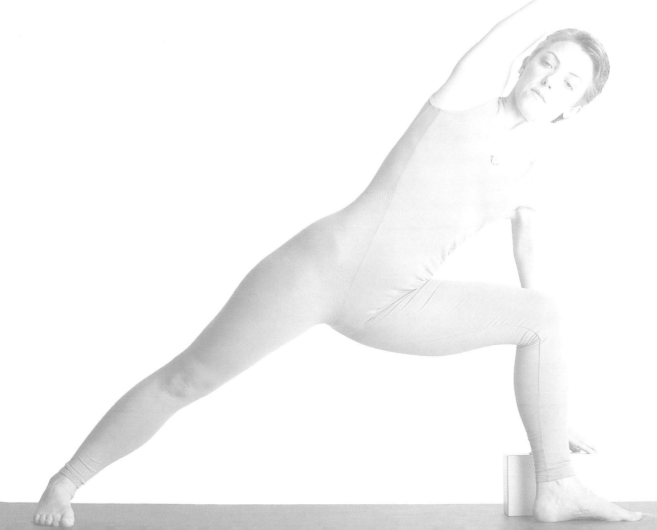

THIS PART OF THE BOOK presents what I call the thirty essential yoga poses (asana) and their variations. As I discuss in Part One, "Beginning with an Ancient Tradition," asana is the most well-known aspect of yoga in the West. Part of a wider philosophy, asana is third limb of Patanjali's classical yoga system. Asana offers time-honored techniques for feeling more at home in your body. When you feel better, you not only enjoy asana practice, but you also have the energy necessary to continue your exploration of the Self, which is the soul of yoga. When you approach the poses with an open mind and loving heart, your journey remains fresh and rewarding as you make the poses your own.

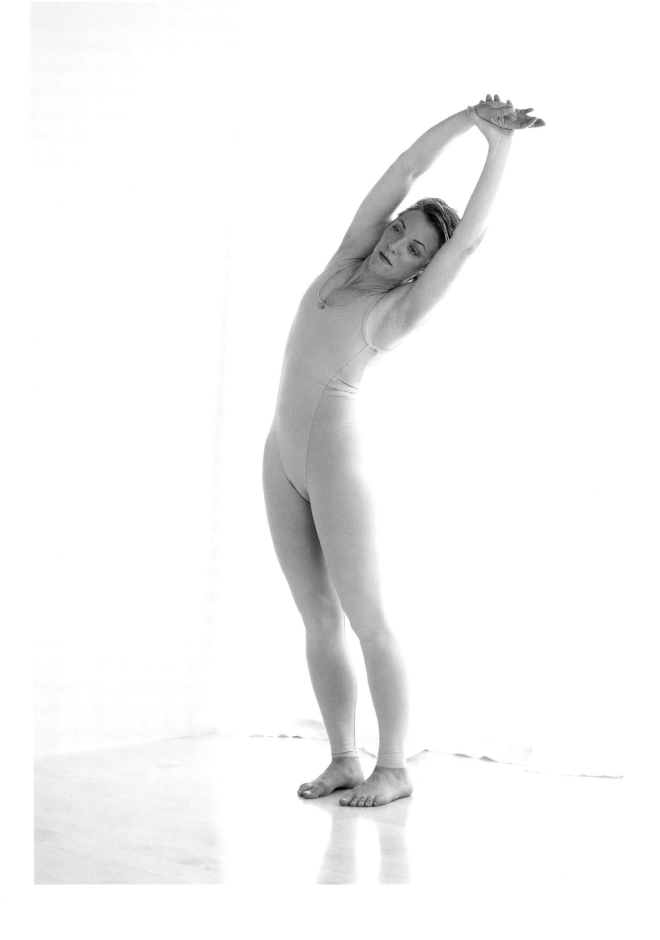

Mountain Pose
Tadasana

1

Mountain Pose (Tadasana) is the foundation pose for all vertical poses. Because standing up seems like such a natural thing, you may not have been taught how to do it well. Paying attention to this pose in your practice and then taking what you learn into your daily life will not only improve your posture, but also may reduce your chance of developing back pain.

The spinal column is arranged in a series of long, graceful curves. To stand well in Mountain Pose, you must allow these curves to assume what anatomists call natural curves. This means that you stand with neither too much nor too little of each curve. Finding, re-establishing, and maintaining these curves whenever possible is what Mountain Pose is all about.

Another powerful lesson that Mountain Pose offers is the experience of "standing on your own two feet" in every way. Learning to center yourself in standing can be done anywhere and anytime: in line at the grocery store, waiting for the bus, or while talking to a friend. Practicing Mountain Pose is one of the easiest ways to integrate your yoga practice into the rest of your life.

I make Mountain Pose more formal by doing it on my nonskid yoga mat as I begin my practice each day. It is a ritual that helps me to make the transition from an informal observing-myself-all-the-time practice to my formal practice of asana.

SEQUENCING. Mountain Pose is unique in that it can be easily inserted between other poses at almost any time during your practice. Often in classes, as well as when you practice at home, this pose is practiced first. But it can also be interspersed between standing poses, as well as used as a finishing and centering moment before Basic Relaxation Pose (Figure 30.1).

BENEFITS. Mountain Pose creates an awareness of your general posture, especially of the spine. It is centering and, when practiced with the eyes closed, can help improve balance.

CAUTIONS. Practice on a firm, level, and nonskid surface. To avoid lightheadedness, do not stand in Mountain Pose for more than one minute, especially if you have low blood pressure.

The Essential Pose *(Figure 1.1)*

PROPS: 1 nonskid mat ✦ 1 mirror

Spread your mat on a firm and level surface, and stand on it with your feet hip-width apart. Begin by looking at your feet: they should point straight ahead. Judge this by drawing an imaginary line from between your second and third toes back toward your ankles. This line should be at a right angle to your inner and outer anklebones, as well as parallel to the line of the other foot. Do not try to make your feet parallel by aligning the inner borders along the arches of your feet. If you do, then your feet will probably be turned out, because the front of your foot is wider than the heel.

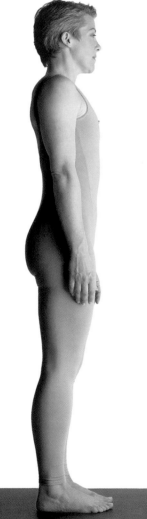

Next, notice the fronts of your top thighs. They are probably pushed forward. Gently bring the weight of your pelvis back. As you do, you will feel your spine lift. If I looked at you from the side, your outer hip would now be in line with your outside anklebone. Glance down to see if this relationship exists, or stand sideways and look in a mirror the first few times that you practice this pose.

Be careful *not* to tuck your tailbone under or flatten your lower back. Although this may be useful exercise while lying down, it does not create healthy or natural spinal curves when standing. You may feel the weight of your body has moved back onto your heel bone, which is where it should be. Do not lock your knees backward.

Draw your shoulder blades down toward your waist just a little, and *then* bring them slightly together. Make your line of vision parallel with the floor. For most of us, this requires a slight dropping of the chin. When you stand like this, your spinal curves will be in neutral and, thus, will be able to bear weight well.

Let your attention rest on your breathing. Can you feel the breath that moves in the back of your body as well as in the front? When you are standing in a balanced and open Mountain Pose, your breath will feel free and unimpeded. If you try to breathe fully when your spine is even slightly rounded, you will notice a definite difficulty.

Stand in Mountain Pose for five to seven slow breaths, but try to practice it whenever you can throughout your day. Remember, Mountain Pose is a great tool for centering yourself without needing to take a more formal meditation posture. To come out of the pose, simply move into an active standing pose, a standing forward bend, whatever pose you are practicing next, or your daily activities.

EXPLORATIONS. From a balanced Mountain Pose, try shifting your weight ever so slightly so that it rests more on one foot. Notice all the changes that happen in your body as you do so. Then shift the weight so that it rests more on the opposite foot. Again, notice what happens. Centralize the weight from the extremes of the two sides. Try this weight-shifting experiment from front to back as well. Observe how standing evenly and balancing on your feet is a dynamic process of adjusting in the moment. What a great thing to remember about life off the mat as well!

FIGURE 1.1

Another way to explore Mountain Pose is to practice with your eyes closed, which is especially useful if you have balance difficulties. Stand in Mountain Pose and look down at the floor at a spot about 3 feet in front of you. Be sure that you do not drop your head as you lower your eyes. Then gradually close your eyes. Keep your breathing soft. Notice the sensations of your body: the feel of your feet pressing against the floor, the sounds that you hear inside and outside the room, and the feel of the rhythm and of your breath. After five breaths, open your eyes and continue with your practice.

VARIATION

PROP: 1 nonskid mat

MOUNTAIN POSE WITH YOUR ARMS OVERHEAD *(Figure 1.2)*. Once you feel truly present in the pose, inhale and stretch your arms overhead, interlocking your fingers. Exhale as you bring your arms down to your sides. Change the interlock and repeat.

ESPECIALLY FOR TEACHERS

PRIMARY FOCUS. Because it is important to create a balanced vertical line of energy in Mountain Pose, look at your student from the side. Draw an imaginary plumb line with your eyes, beginning with the student's outer ear. That line should pass down through the center of the shoulder, hip, knee, and ankle joints.

PRIMARY ADJUSTMENT. Most people in Western cultures habitually stand with the pelvis pushed forward. Suggest to your student that he gently move the pelvis back. You can check if the student is in an aligned Mountain Pose by the following test. Ask your student for permission to touch him. When you receive this permission, stand behind the student and then place your hands on the tops of his shoulders, your right hand on his right shoulder and your left on his left. Firmly press straight down with about 8 to 10 pounds of pressure. (Do not attempt this if the student is suffering from diagnosed disc disease, osteoporosis of the spinal column, or chronic back pain.)

If the student's spine is aligned with the natural curves intact, then he will be able to hold this weight easily. If the student sways under your pressure, check the plumb line again. Usually asking the student to move the pelvis back and to make the shoulder blades vertical will allow him to hold your pressure the second time. When the student is aligned, your downward pressure will feel good, and will not cause your student to move or buckle. You can use this simple test in class while other students are practicing the pose. It also makes a dramatic presentation. Be sure to ask and receive permission to touch each student, each time.

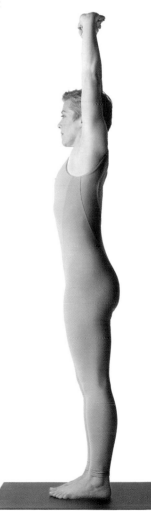

FIGURE 1.2

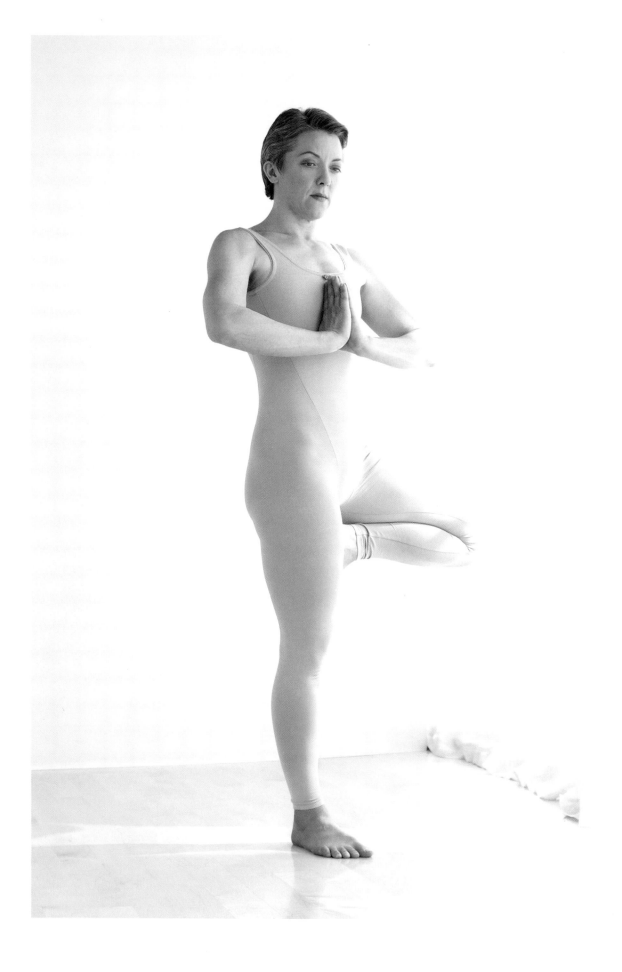

Tree Pose
Vrksasana

2

TREE POSE (Vrksasana) presents you with the challenge of balancing on one foot. As a child, you probably could stand on one foot and balance by the age of five. Doctors sometimes use the ability to perform this task as a measure of neurological maturity. But as an adult you may have lost this acuity of balance, partly out of neglect. Practice Tree Pose not only to improve your balance, but also to increase your ability to focus.

SEQUENCING. Practice Tree Pose directly after Mountain Pose (Figure 1.1).

BENEFITS. Tree Pose teaches balance and focus, and is fun for students of all ages. It helps to strengthen the muscles of the supporting foot.

CAUTIONS. Practice Tree Pose on a firm, level, and nonskid surface. Do not attempt this pose if you are feeling dizzy. It not recommended for women who are more than six months pregnant.

The Essential Pose *(Figure 2.1)*

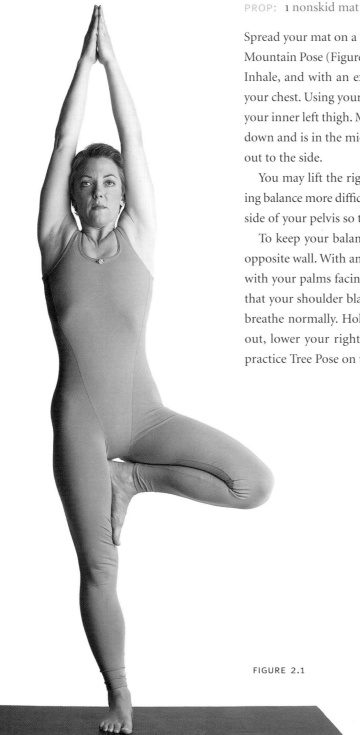

FIGURE 2.1

PROP: 1 nonskid mat

Spread your mat on a firm and level surface, and stand on it in Mountain Pose (Figure 1.1). Shift your weight onto your left leg. Inhale, and with an exhalation, bend your right knee toward your chest. Using your right hand, place your foot at the top of your inner left thigh. Make sure that your right foot is pointing down and is in the middle of your thigh. Turn your right knee out to the side.

You may lift the right side of the pelvis up too much, making balance more difficult. As much as is possible, drop the right side of your pelvis so that it is level from side to side.

To keep your balance, focus your vision on a point on the opposite wall. With an inhalation, stretch your arms overhead, with your palms facing each other and elbows straight. Lift so that your shoulder blades move up. Keep your throat soft and breathe normally. Hold the pose for several breaths. To come out, lower your right leg and resume Mountain Pose. Then practice Tree Pose on the opposite side.

EXPLORATIONS. Perhaps one of the hardest things to achieve in life is balance. Learning to work, play, rest, and serve others in proportions that enhance your health and that of others is an art. Tree Pose explores the physical balance that is created by focusing on just this pose in this moment.

When you practice it, focus on your concentration spot on the wall, your breath, or the sensations of the moment. Healthy living springs, in part, from your ability to be fully present and do one thing at a time and do it completely.

Another way of exploring balance in Tree Pose is to close the eyes. Balance is both a visual and a kinesthetic experience. You might use visual cues to help you balance but ignore the contributions made by the kinesthetic, or the body position, sense. After you have lifted your arms overhead in Tree Pose, slowly close your eyes. Notice how the ankle of your supporting foot immediately begins to move back and forth in an attempt to keep you balanced. You have removed the visual cues to your balance and thus must rely more on your body's sense of itself in space. Do not hold your breath when you are focusing on balancing in the pose. Try to take three breaths before opening your eyes and repeating on the other side.

Explore Tree Pose with clarity and commitment, and take this balance into your life.

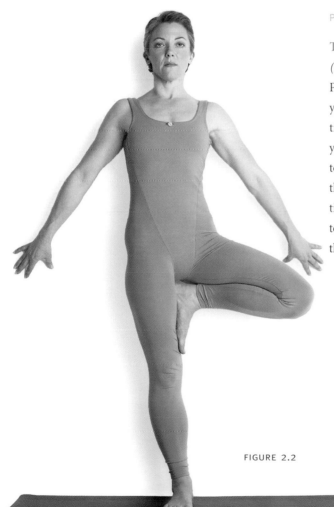

FIGURE 2.2

VARIATIONS

PROPS: 1 nonskid mat ✦ 1 wall

TREE POSE WITH YOUR HANDS AT THE WALL (*Figure 2.2*). If you cannot balance in Tree Pose, try it near a smooth wall. Stand with your back about 6 inches from the wall. Practice Tree Pose as previously described, but use your hands behind you for support. Lightly touch your fingers on the wall and then take them away briefly so that you do not lean continuously on the wall. This will help you learn to balance more quickly than if you hold onto the wall the whole time.

TREE POSE WITH YOUR HANDS IN NAMASTE *(Figure 2.3)*. Once you have positioned your foot on your thigh in Tree Pose and feel balanced, try this variation with the arms. Instead of stretching them overhead, bring your palms together in front of your heart. Make sure that the edges of your palms and all the length of your fingers touch firmly but gently and that your fingers point upward. This shape of the hands is the Prayer Position, or Namaste, which is often seen in yoga classes. The word *namaste* comes from the Sanskrit word *namas*, which is translated "salutations to you." This gesture expresses respect and honor for yourself and others. Breathe normally in the pose, and stay for three breaths before repeating it on the other side.

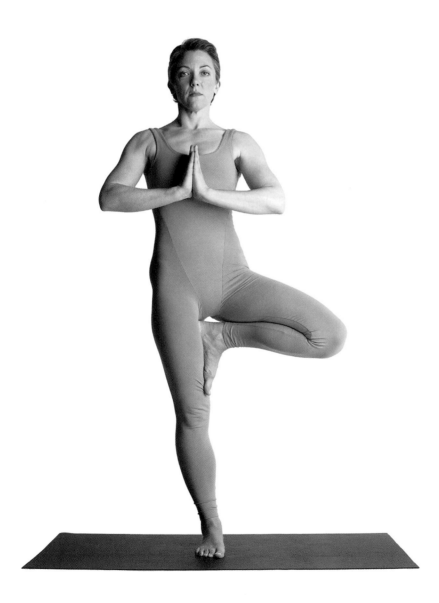

FIGURE 2.3

ESPECIALLY FOR TEACHERS

PRIMARY FOCUS. Students usually think that Tree Pose is about balance only and overlook the need for symmetry in the pose. One way to help them create symmetry as well as enhance their balance is to remind them of a useful idea: drop the pelvis *down* on the bent-knee side while lifting *up* from the arm on that same side. This sense of dropping down with the pelvis and lifting up on the same side with the arm helps to create stability.

PRIMARY ADJUSTMENT. If the student is having a hard time with keeping the foot in place, have him or her experiment with the placement of the heel. Although it should be placed in the middle of the opposite thigh, some students find it useful to lower the foot closer to the knee. Others even like placing their foot on the opposite inner knee. Encourage experimentation. This will help the student own his or her practice, which is the best thing that we can teach our students.

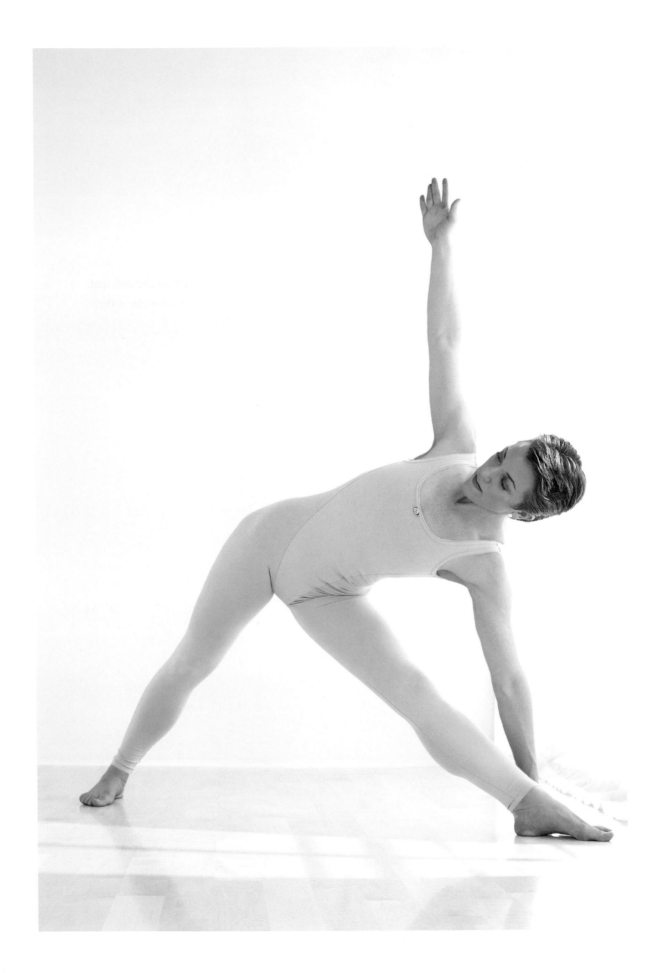

Extended Triangle Pose
Utthita Trikonasana

3

Extended Triangle Pose (Utthita Trikonasana) is taught as a basic pose in virtually all the different approaches to asana, whether the style is slow or vigorous. In fact, most yoga students consider it their favorite standing pose. Commonly referred to as Triangle Pose, it provides challenges for the beginning student, as well as for the experienced practitioner.

For the beginner, the joys of Extended Triangle Pose are experienced as the hip joints and chest open, and as the legs stretch and strengthen. For the more experienced student, it reminds him or her also of the balance of opposites that is the heart of yoga philosophy: the strength and power of the legs in contrast to the lifting and soaring of the back and arms. Regardless of your level of practice, Extended Triangle Pose is an important standing pose and it will continue to provide you with new insights for years to come.

SEQUENCING. Practice Extended Triangle Pose after Mountain Pose (Figure 1.1). Occasionally, I like to intersperse this pose between other standing poses. When I do, Extended Triangle Pose becomes a touchstone to gauge the effects of other poses. In addition, the effects of Extended Triangle Pose become clearer. Each time it feels a little different, and I feel a little more open. This way of practicing is appropriate for experienced beginners as well as more advanced students.

At other times, I begin my practice with Extended Triangle Pose, putting it even before Mountain Pose. Varying the order of my practice increases my perception of the effects of both Mountain Pose and Extended Triangle Pose, and helps to keep my practice alive and interesting.

BENEFITS. Extended Triangle Pose improves the balance, stretches the hamstring muscles, increases the flexibility of the hip joints, strengthens the front thigh muscles, and stretches the back.

CAUTIONS. Extended Triangle Pose is not recommended during the menstrual period, or when your balance may be shaky, such as when you are recovering from the flu. If the latter is the case, then practice with your back to the wall for added support. If you are in the last six weeks of pregnancy, practice with your back against the wall for added balance. Avoid this or any other pose if it increases lower back pain.

The Essential Pose *(Figure 3.1)*

PROP: 1 nonskid mat

Spread your mat on a firm and level surface, and stand on it in Mountain Pose (Figure 1.1). Separate your feet approximately 4 to 4½ feet apart. This distance for all standing poses is individual and depends on two things. The first of these variables is the length of your legs. As a general rule, the longer your legs, the wider the distance. This pose gets its name from the triangular shape that is formed by your legs. Look down and determine if this triangle is an equilateral one. If not, then step your feet wider apart or closer together to create this shape.

Second, your suppleness and balance will influence how far apart your feet will be. Do not place them at a distance that either compromises your stability or creates a strong stretch on your inner knees when you turn your feet. If either of these happens, bring your feet closer together. You can increase the length of your stance over time.

Turn your left foot inward, so that your toes point about halfway toward your right foot. Turn your right foot out so that your right toes point away from you. If you drew a line from your right heel to your left foot, it would intersect the middle of your left arch. Most people do not turn the front foot (in this case, the right foot) out enough, so take a moment to make sure that your foot is indeed turning out to 90 degrees.

Inhale as you lift your arms out to your sides and to shoulder height. Exhale as you stretch them out fully. Continue to breathe normally. Make sure that your right kneecap is turning toward your right little toe. Do not let it turn inward, because this movement may stress the knee joint.

It is critical that you turn your knee out so that the front leg is in alignment, that is, so that the center of your kneecap is pointing over your outer foot and is not rolling in.

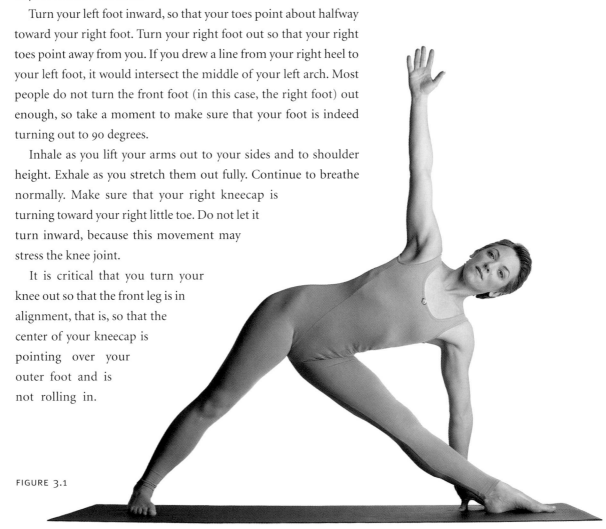

FIGURE 3.1

The entire leg is meant to rotate externally, or turn out strongly. If your torso turns in the direction of the leg, then that is fine. The priority here is the alignment of the front leg, especially the knee joint. It is important that the quadriceps femoris are active, which has the effect of lifting the kneecaps. If you find this action mysterious, then be sure to read "Primary Focus" in the section entitled "Especially for Teachers," which follows.

Inhale and as you exhale, stretch out to the side, elongating your spine to the right and swinging your hips to the left. Keep exhaling the entire time that you are moving. Place your right hand on your right lower shin or higher. Remember, the emphasis here is on stretching *out* and not on going *down*. If this action seems difficult, then try the variation called Extended Triangle Pose with Your Hand on a Block (Figure 3.2).

Extended Triangle Pose is a movement that comes from the hip joints. When you practice it this way, your rib cage will be parallel to the floor, not rounding upward. Remember, this is not a traditional side stretch: instead, the stretch is brought into the legs and hip joints. Take care to drop your ribs, even if this means that you need to bring your hand up higher on your leg.

Once you are in the pose, keep your knees straight and your front thigh muscles contracting to give strength and support to the knee joints. Stretch your left arm straight up toward the ceiling. It is easy to let it stretch back past the vertical. To counteract this tendency, put your emphasis on turning your belly upward. Position your head so that you are looking straight ahead, not up; soften your eyes and breathe regularly. Hold the pose for several breaths. Come up with an inhalation, and repeat on the other side.

EXPLORATION. Every yoga pose involves all of you, even though it may seemingly focus on a specific part of your body. Extended Triangle Pose is no exception. Once you are in the pose, stretch out through both arms and both legs. Firmly press down through the back leg, and roll the front leg out as you press it down as well. Reaching upward may seem more obvious, but reaching and stretching down is equally important.

Expand your body out along the lines of your limbs in all directions from your center like a starfish. Turn your belly upward. At the same time that you ask your body to stretch outward, invite your mind to roll inward like a wave receding from the shore. Enjoy the contrast of an extroverted body and an introverted mind.

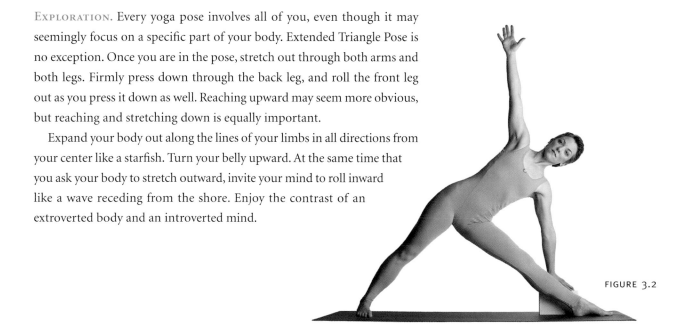

FIGURE 3.2

VARIATIONS

PROPS: 1 nonskid mat ✦ 1 block
1 wall

EXTENDED TRIANGLE POSE WITH YOUR HAND ON A BLOCK *(Figure 3.2)*. When learning Extended Triangle Pose, it may be difficult or even uncomfortable to rest your supporting hand on your shin or ankle. Try this variation. After you have placed your feet in the wide stance for Extended Triangle Pose, put a block beside your outer ankle. After stretching out, place your fingers on the block. The support makes it easier for you to enjoy your pose.

Even if you have been practicing for years, it can be interesting to use a block every now and then. Paradoxically, the block *lessens* the stretch. When this happens, you will experience new sensations, which can be a focus of attention. As you will discover, experimenting with a prop can help to keep a pose fresh.

EXTENDED TRIANGLE POSE WITH YOUR ARM OVERHEAD *(Figure 3.3)*. When Extended Triangle Pose feels like a familiar friend, you may want to try this variation. Once you have stretched to the side, exhale and move your top arm so that it is in a diagonal line with your torso and back leg. Enjoy the feeling of stretch from your back foot up and out through your fingers.

EXTENDED TRIANGLE POSE WITH YOUR ARM BEHIND YOUR WAIST *(Figure 3.4)* Another interesting variation of Extended Triangle Pose is to wrap your top arm around your back waist. Do this movement on an exhalation when you feel settled and balanced in the posture. Once your arm is wrapped around your back, then turn your elbow back to help open the chest a little more. Remember to breathe.

EXTENDED TRIANGLE POSE, FACING THE WALL *(Figure 3.5)*. To enhance your ability to open your hip joints and chest in Extended Triangle Pose, practice this variation. Place your nonskid mat so that the edge of your mat is just touching the wall. Stand on your mat about 1 foot away from the wall, and face the wall. Move into Extended Triangle Pose and then put your fingertips lightly on the wall with your hands placed

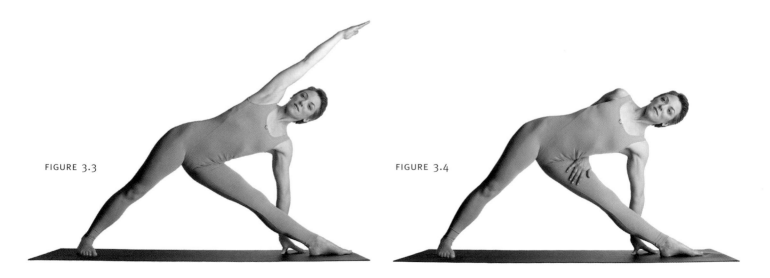

FIGURE 3.3

FIGURE 3.4

slightly wider than your shoulders. With an exhalation, push your fingers against the wall and use that leverage to rotate your chest upward. Be careful not to lean into the wall. If you do, then you will lose the leverage necessary to rotate upward.

ESPECIALLY FOR TEACHERS

PRIMARY FOCUS. Even when a student has been practicing for many years, it can still be difficult for him or her to remember how to use the feet and legs. The weight on the front foot should be distributed on the ball of the foot with a little more weight on the ball of the big toe. This is balanced by placing a little more weight on the outer heel. When the student presses both these places equally, the foot will remain balanced between a dynamic and stable state.

Sometimes a student has problems translating the thought of straightening the legs into an actual contraction of the quadriceps muscles in the front thigh. To help this student, try this simple exercise. Have your student sit down on the floor, with the legs straight out in front and the quadriceps relaxed. Then ask your student to reach down with one hand and gently wiggle his or her kneecap from side to side. This should be easy to do and painless.

Now ask your student to contract his or her quadriceps. This is easy to do if the student *imagines* lifting his or her leg off the floor an inch. The student should then try to move the kneecap from side to side. This is impossible if these muscles are contracting, because the quadriceps tendon presses the kneecap down into the leg and disallows any sideways movement of the kneecap. When I show a student what it means to truly contract the quadriceps femoris, it is often easier for him or her to do it in Extended Triangle Pose.

PRIMARY ADJUSTMENT. To help your student understand how to drop the top ribs in the pose, try this aid. Stand behind your student as she practices Extended Triangle Pose to the right. After asking and receiving permission to touch her, gently hold the student's left wrist with your right hand. Place your left fingertips lightly but firmly on your student's left top ribs. Ask your student to exhale and simultaneously press down softly on her ribs as you gently pull up on her wrist. This should cause the student's ribs to drop down toward the floor. Then quietly ask the student to repeat this movement on her own so that you can be sure that she understands what you were suggesting.

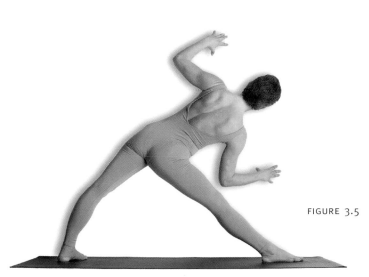

FIGURE 3.5

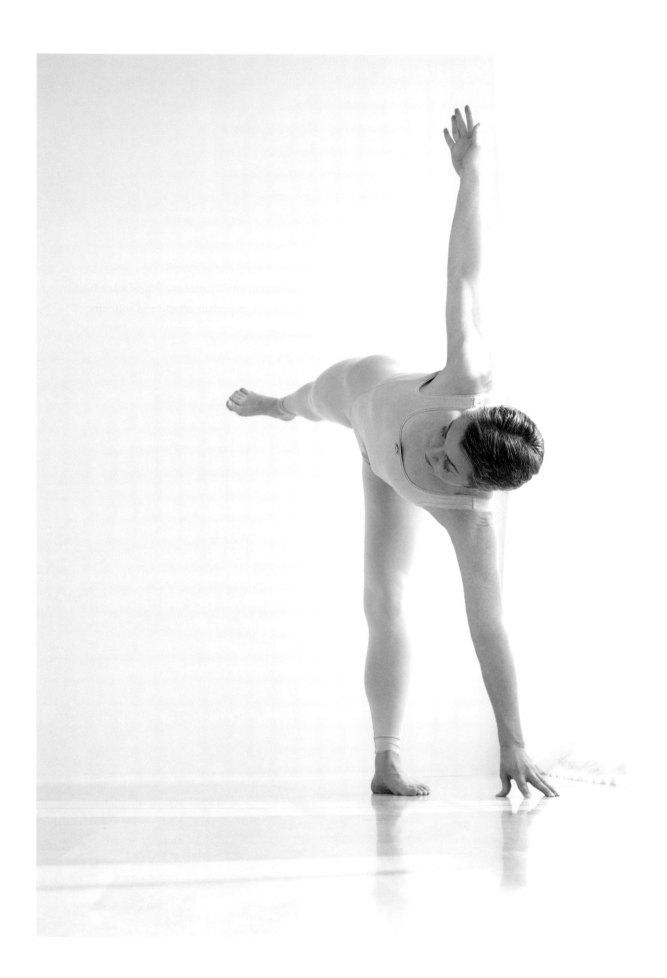

Half-Moon Pose
Ardha Chandrasana

4

COMBINING BALANCE AND STRETCH, Half-Moon Pose (Ardha Chandrasana) partakes of the cool radiance of the moon in the midst of the heat of active standing poses. It is especially effective in softening and opening the belly. Remember the soaring feeling of Half-Moon Pose when you are stuck in the doldrums of life.

SEQUENCING. Half-Moon Pose naturally emerges from Extended Triangle Pose (Figure 3.1).

BENEFITS. As you stand, poised on one leg like a dancer, Half-Moon Pose improves your balance, stretches the hamstring muscles in the backs of your thighs, increases the flexibility of your hip joints, strengthens your front thigh muscles, and stretches out your back. It gives you confidence as you learn to balance and open at the same time.

CAUTIONS. Half-Moon Pose is not recommended during the menstrual period, or when your balance may be shaky, such as when you are recovering from the flu. If the latter is the case, then practice with your back to the wall for added support. If you are a woman who is five months pregnant or more, practice with your back at the wall and a block under your hand.

The Essential Pose *(Figure 4.1)*

PROP: 1 nonskid mat

Spread your mat on a firm and level surface, and stand on it in Mountain Pose (Figure 1.1). Separate your feet about 4 to 4½ feet apart, lift your arms to the sides, and turn your feet as for Extended Triangle Pose (Figure 3.1). Then narrow your stance just slightly. Come into Extended Triangle Pose to the right.

Exhale as you bend your right knee, and place your right fingertips on the floor just beyond, and to the side of, your toes. Try not to keep your chest lifted. Inhale, and as you exhale, move your torso up, out,

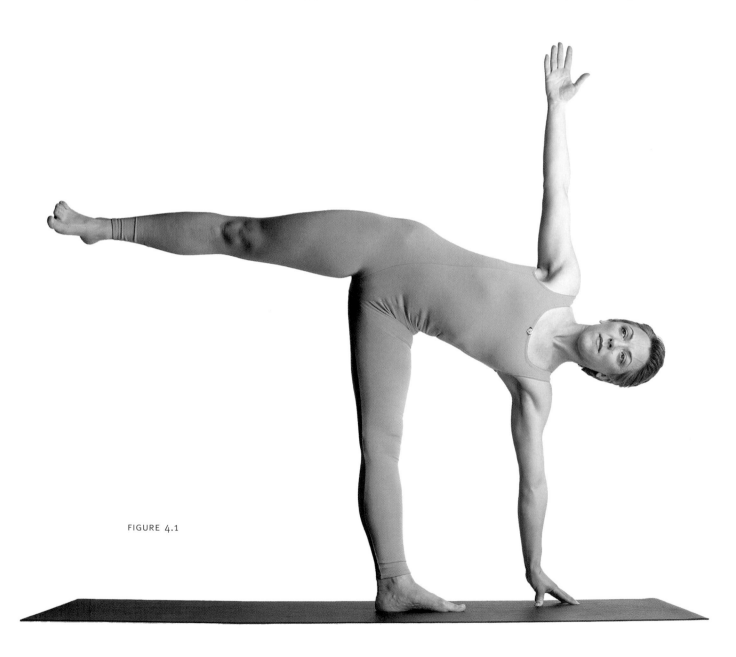

FIGURE 4.1

and over your foot, straightening your right leg and lifting your left leg so that it is horizontal to the floor. Move your fingers forward on the floor as is necessary to keep your balance. Think of the back leg as the source of stability–your anchor–in the pose. This will allow you to rotate your trunk upward and thus to open more.

Continue to breathe normally and open your chest toward the heavens. Stretch out in all directions, through both arms and legs.

Hold the pose for several breaths. Come out of the pose by stretching back with the top leg as you bend your front knee. Place your left foot back where it was when you started. Now straighten your front leg into Extended Triangle Pose. Hold Extended Triangle Pose for one breath, and come up on an inhalation. Practice the pose on the other side.

EXPLORATION. Finding your balance in Half-Moon Pose is not something that happens at the end of the pose, but rather at the very beginning. It comes, in large part, from the position that you establish with your front foot.

You might move your supporting foot in the process of coming up into the pose. This usually manifests as a slight inward rotation of the front foot. The intention of this movement is, no doubt, to create more stability, but it actually creates less. This occurs because an inward rotation of the thighbone causes less surface area to touch in the hip joint, which is made up of the pelvis and thighbone. The less surface area that touches, the less stable the pose.

Ironically, what you do to create stability in the pose is the very thing that creates *instability*. Remember, practice Half-Moon Pose with your front foot firmly planted in the position that you establish at the outset. It seems that in this pose, as in life, balance is something that you *maintain*, not something that you *create*.

VARIATIONS

PROPS: 1 nonskid mat   ✦   1 block
1 wall

HALF-MOON POSE WITH YOUR HAND ON A BLOCK *(Figure 4.2)*. You may find it difficult to reach the floor in the completed pose. If this happens, stand on your mat, near the back edge. Place your block where your hand will be in the completed pose, that is, behind the mat and slightly forward. Come into Extended Triangle Pose, reach out with your front arm, and place your hand on the block. Slide the block along the floor until it is directly under your shoulder. Lean on the block firmly. To come down, as you lower your back leg and bend the front one, slide the block back with you. Let go of the block as you come up into Extended Triangle Pose. Repeat to the other side.

HALF-MOON POSE AT THE WALL AND WITH A BLOCK *(Figure 4.3)*. If you are finding it a challenge to balance, then take your mat to the wall and place it with the long side parallel to the wall. Place your block as in the previous variation, and turn your back to the wall. Come into the pose and lean your back against the wall. Use the block to support your front arm.

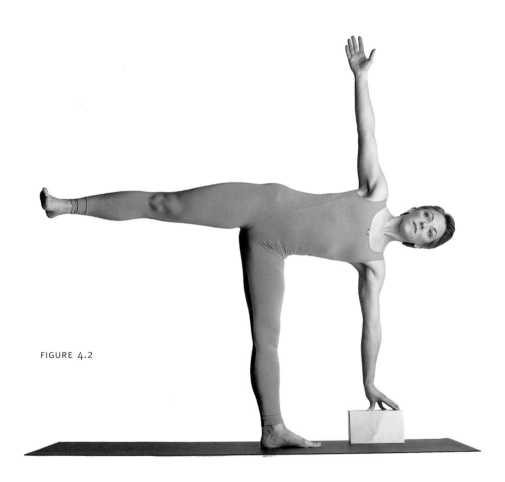

FIGURE 4.2

ESPECIALLY FOR TEACHERS

PRIMARY FOCUS. A child is taught to be goal oriented: ace a good the test, make the team, or win the game. As the child matures, his approach to life may remain the same, with only the goals changing. Perhaps he comes to seek fame, money, or some other expression of status. His approach to yoga may be no different: he wants to *do* the pose, he wants to *get* the pose. It doesn't occur to him to be interested in what he can learn during the *process* of moving into and out of a pose. Remind your students to stay focused during the transition of going into and coming out of Half-Moon Pose. For example, ask them to bring awareness to the physical sensations they experience during the transition, or suggest that after coming out of the pose they reflect upon their thoughts and feelings about the transition. Practicing and teaching yoga means that you bring *awareness to the process*, not just the end point.

PRIMARY ADJUSTMENT. A student often comes into Half-Moon Pose, completely straights the supporting leg, and *then* tries to open the chest. Suggest that your student open the chest *while* coming into the pose. To do this, when the student is two-thirds of the way up, have him or her turn and open the chest, and *then* straighten the lower leg. Practicing this way is physically and mentally powerful. Physically, the student will find that there is actually more opening created. Mentally, it will reinforce the experience of remaining open in the midst of life as it happens, and not waiting until everything is *done* or *perfect* before finding the courage to open.

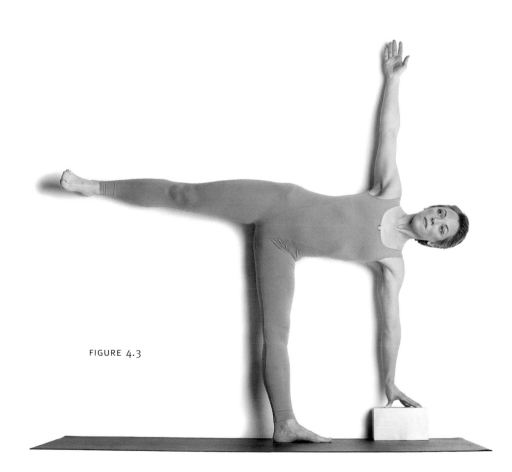

FIGURE 4.3

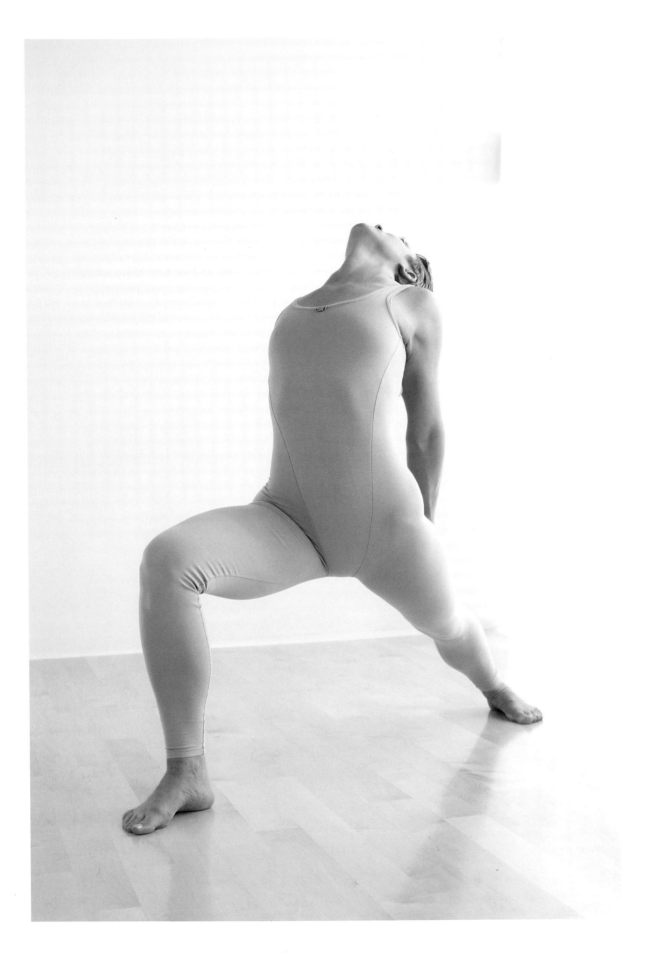

Warrior I Pose
Virabhadrasana I

5

THE COURAGE of the warrior is a theme of both Western and Eastern literature, and has been so since time out of mind. Consider the heroic deeds of the maid of Orléans, whose startling poise and bravery in leading French soldiers into battle are portrayed in playwright George Bernard Shaw's *Saint Joan*. He wrote this masterpiece in 1923, just four years after the girl-warrior was declared a saint. Virabhadra is an incarnation of Siva, the god of destruction and regeneration in the Hindu sacred triad. He strikes a formidable pose with his one thousand heads, one thousand eyes, and one thousand feet. He wears a tiger skin, and is armed with one thousand clubs. Siva is commemorated in Warrior I Pose, which requires focus, strength, and power.

SEQUENCING. Warrior I Pose naturally follows Extended Triangle Pose (Figure 3.1) and leads to Warrior II Pose (Figure 6.1).

BENEFITS. Warrior I Pose strengthens the quadriceps muscles of the front leg, stretches the calf of the back leg, and improves shoulder and upper back flexibility.

CAUTIONS. Warrior I Pose is not recommended during the menstrual period, or when your balance may be shaky, such as when you are recovering from the flu. If the latter is the case, then practice the pose with your back to the wall for added support. Avoid this pose if your knees are swollen or painful, and during pregnancy from about six months. Do not practice this pose if it exacerbates existing back pain.

The Essential Pose *(Figure 5.1)*

PROP: 1 nonskid mat

Spread your mat on a firm and level surface, and stand on it in Mountain Pose (Figure 1.1). Separate your feet about 4 to 4½ feet apart as for Extended Triangle Pose (Figure 3.1). Lift your arms out to the sides, and turn your feet to the right. To review these points, see page 26.

Inhale as you enthusiastically stretch your arms overhead. Continue to breathe normally. Lift your chest and, with an exhalation, turn your torso to face your right leg. Firmly press your back heel into the floor. With the next exhalation, bend your front knee to square your thigh and lower leg. Initially, you may not be able to get down into the right angle, but this will improve with practice. Your back leg should remain straight and firm and your breathing normal throughout the pose. Keep your line of vision parallel to the floor, and your face and throat relaxed.

Hold the pose for several breaths, and come up on an inhalation. Turn to the front with an exhalation, lowering your arms to your sides. Repeat to the other side.

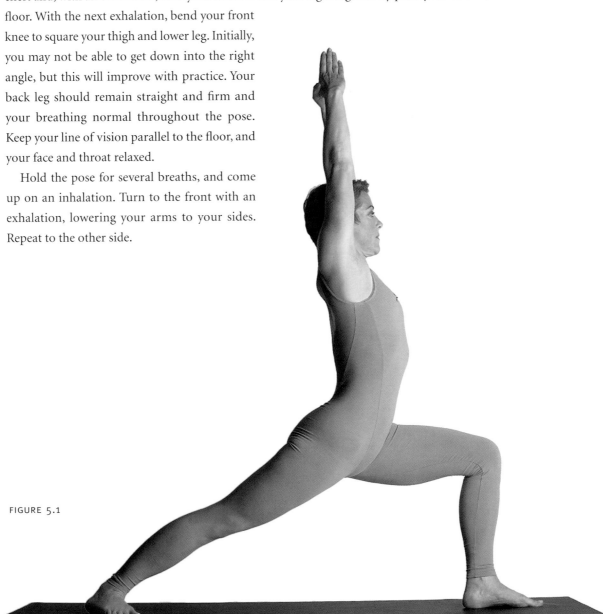

FIGURE 5.1

EXPLORATION. One of the greatest challenges of Warrior I Pose is learning to turn completely toward the front leg. Focusing on three points can help. First, make sure that your back foot is well turned toward the front one. Experiment with turning it in even a little more, and see if this movement helps you rotate your torso.

Next, focus on turning from your hips. Bring the left hip forward when practicing to the right side (of course, the opposite is true when practicing to the left). Try to bring your hip forward so that both hipbones are level and in the same plane.

Finally, you may tend to understretch the arm on the side of the body where the leg is back. To counteract this, bring your left shoulder into the turn, and combine this with stretching your left arm a little more than your right. Even though you are stretching more from the left, this will actually produce an even shape of the arms.

VARIATIONS

PROP: 2 nonskid mats

WARRIOR I POSE WITH A ROLLED MAT UNDER YOUR BACK FOOT (*Figure 5.2*). To avoid sliding and for stability in this variation, first stand on a nonskid mat that has been spread out as usual for standing poses.

You may find it difficult to keep the back heel down, or if you do try to keep it down, then you may sacrifice the amount of turning that is required to practice with stability. Remedy this by *firmly* rolling another mat and placing it under your back heel before you begin the pose. This variation will help to give you support as you learn to simultaneously lengthen your back lower leg and turn your torso.

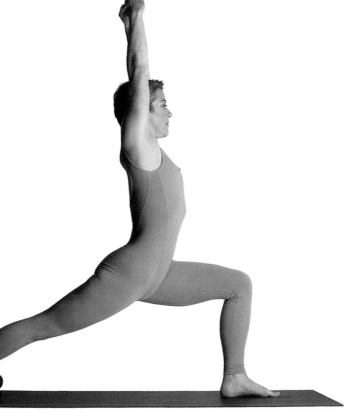

FIGURE 5.2

WARRIOR I POSE WITH YOUR HEAD BACK *(Figure 5.3). Do not practice this variation if you have problems with your neck or a tendency to get dizzy.* If you have practiced this pose for a few months, then you may want to tilt your head back after you bend your front knee. This movement is usually accompanied by bringing your arms together at the palms, so that they are in line with the front of the face. If you try this, then remember to keep the arms perpendicular to the floor, and the head and neck free as they arch back.

Do *not* drop the head by taking the chin forward. Instead, tilt your head back by lifting your chest and then letting the neck go back. Practicing this way will let the head hang easily. Keep your gaze soft and your breathing regular. To come out of the pose, lift your head with an inhalation. Exhale as you straighten the front leg. Then turn your feet and torso forward, and repeat to the other side.

ESPECIALLY FOR TEACHERS

PROPS: 1 or 2 nonskid mats   ✦   1 wall

PRIMARY FOCUS. As with all poses in which the knee is bent and weight bearing, attention should be given to the student's front knee. Make sure that the kneecap is directly over the little toe when the knee is bent. Also ensure that the student's hip joint stays in line with the forward heel.

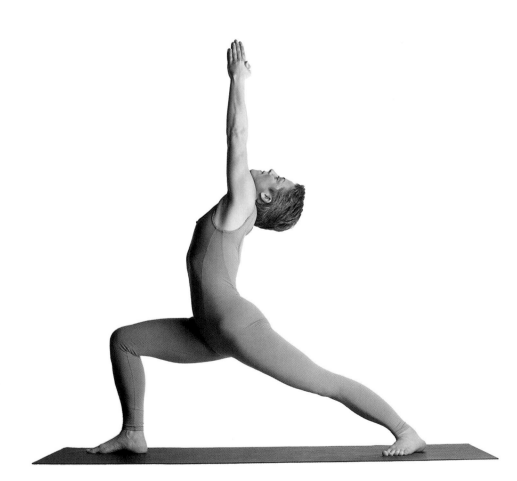

FIGURE 5.3

Warrior I Pose includes a slight back bending movement, so do not worry if an arch appears in the lower back. This arch will be apparent especially when the student stretches his or her arms overhead. Encourage the student to keep the back leg straight, and the weight distributed evenly between the legs. The torso should be held upright, and the chest should be open. These points of awareness will help the student practice the pose in an enjoyable and powerful way.

PRIMARY ADJUSTMENT. When a student stretches the arms overhead, he or she may not fully stretch them. If this happens, then suggest that the student lift the shoulder blades as part of the stretch of the arms. This movement is part of the gleno-humeral rhythm of shoulder joints; it is natural and necessary to a full range of movement. Remember, this movement should not be accompanied by tension in the throat, but by muscular action in the back and shoulders.

To help the student understand this movement more fully, have him or her practice it with only one arm lifted. Alternatively, this movement can be learned at the wall. Have the student place the hands on the wall, about halfway between shoulder and waist height, and bend forward. Then, with the hands still on the wall, the student should push away from the wall, allowing the sides of the ribs to move back *and* the shoulder blades to move toward the wall. Have the student repeat this movement several times. Practicing this way will help the student feel what the shoulder blade movement is like before trying it in the pose.

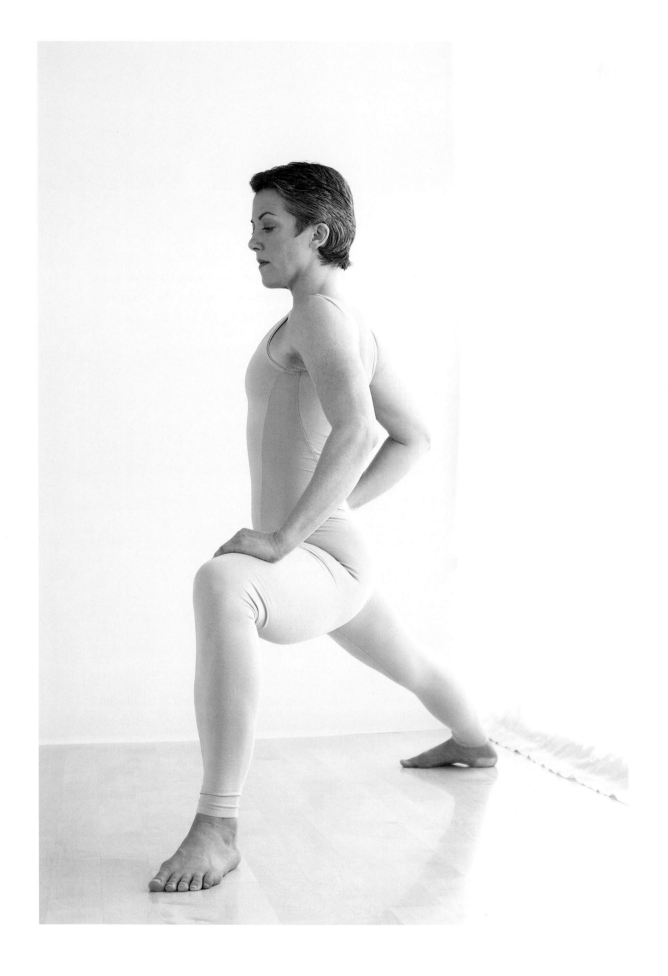

Warrior II Pose
Virabhadrasana II

6

THE ETHICAL DILEMMA of the warrior is explored in the Bhagavadgita (c. 500–300 B.C.E.), a Sanskrit epic that reports the battlefield dialogue between Prince Arjuna and the god-man Krisna. The prince is an archer and the god man is his charioteer. Riddled with doubt, fear, and indecision as he prepares for battle, Arjuna opens to self-discovery through Krisna's counsel. Translated as "The Lord's Song," this seven hundred–stanza poem charts a course of selfless right action, even in battle.

Arjuna is each of us, and his battlefield is a metaphor for our lives. Through asana practice, we can understand his (and our) dilemma. Warrior II Pose (Virabhadrasana II) echoes the powerful lunge of the archer, and underscores the importance of attention, strength, and courage as we take up asana practice. It challenges us to contain several actions at once: to stretch backward and forward with the arms at the same time *and* keep the torso still. As we learn to maintain this dynamic balance on the mat, we can explore this state when *off* the mat. Like Arjuna, we *can* be present to what is happening in our lives. Through awareness, we *can* open ourselves to the choice to respond with clarity when in doubt, with courage when fearful, and with appropriate boundaries when indecisive.

SEQUENCING. Practice Warrior II Pose after Extended Triangle Pose (Figure 3.1) or Warrior I Pose (Figure 5.1). Follow it with Extended Side-Angle Stretch Pose (Figure 7.1).

BENEFITS. Warrior II Pose strengthens most of your leg muscles, including the hamstrings and quadriceps, and stretches the adductor muscles. In addition, it mobilizes your hip joints and improves their function.

CAUTIONS. Warrior II Pose is not recommended during the menstrual period or when your balance may be shaky, such as when you are recovering from the flu. If the latter is the case, then practice with your back to the wall for added support. Avoid this pose if your knees are swollen or painful, and after the sixth month of pregnancy.

The Essential Pose *(Figure 6.1)*

PROPS   1 nonskid mat   ✦   1 mirror

Spread your mat on a firm and level surface, and stand on it in Mountain Pose (Figure 1.1). As in Extended Triangle Pose (Figure 3.1), separate your feet about 4 to 4½ feet apart, lift your arms out to the sides, and turn your feet to the right. To refresh your understanding of these points, see page 26.

The priority in this pose is the alignment of the front leg, especially the knee joint. It is critical that you turn your knee out so that the front leg is in alignment. It is permissible to turn your torso slightly toward the front leg. Keep the quadriceps active by extending through your heel, which will have the effect of lifting your kneecaps. If you find this action mysterious, then be sure to read the "Primary Focus" section, under "Especially for Teachers," in Extended Triangle Pose (Figure 3.1).

As you exhale, bend your right knee so that your kneecap points directly over your right little toe. Take special care that your knee stays back and does not move forward over the arch of your foot. Keep your back knee straight. Stretch back through your left arm so that your torso remains vertical and posi-

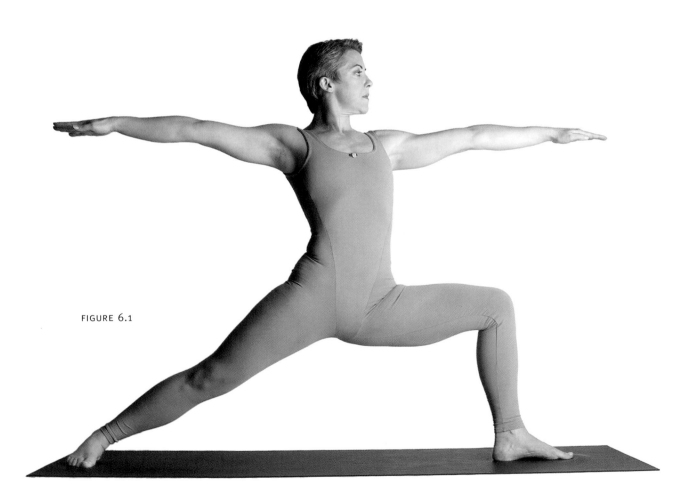

FIGURE 6.1

tioned over the middle of your legs. Do not let it incline forward over your front leg. Turn your head to look over your front leg. Keep your line of vision parallel to the floor, and do not tilt your head to the side.

As you bend your right knee, exhale and square your front thigh and lower leg. You may want to try this pose in front of a full-length mirror to see what it feels like to create this shape. Most people do not go down far enough in this movement, but be careful not to push yourself past your ability. The true practice of yoga is about discovering your limit, remaining present with that limit, and not pushing past it. Remember, pushing can lead to injury.

When you bend your knee, make sure that your torso does not turn toward that knee, but keep your chest and belly looking straight ahead. There should be no rotation in your pelvis toward the bent leg. Your pelvis should remain in a neutral position as much as possible. Once you are in the pose, continue to breathe naturally. Hold the pose for three to five breaths, and come up on an inhalation. Repeat to the other side.

EXPLORATION. This pose appears to be about moving forward over the front leg as you go into the pose. But it is also about remaining still. In order to create a balance between *moving forward* and having the sense of *going nowhere* at the same time, it is important that you think of moving in two directions at once as you bend your knee. This means that as you stretch forward, you also stretch back with equal awareness.

Imagine that the front arm represents the future and the back arm the past. When you equalize the stretch between this future and past, you are focused on remaining in the present. Learning to be present with the pose and the moment are the root of yoga.

VARIATION

PROPS: 1 nonskid mat   ✦   1 wall

WARRIOR II POSE WITH YOUR BACK FOOT AGAINST THE WALL (*Figure 6.2*). Position your mat with the short end against the wall. Place your left foot against the wall, so that your little toe and the length of the outside of your foot are in contact with the wall. This time you are not turning your back foot in.

Follow the instructions in "The Essential Pose," pressing your back foot against the wall throughout. This action will help you develop awareness of your back leg even though you cannot see it. Inhale as you come up, and repeat to the other side.

ESPECIALLY FOR TEACHERS

PRIMARY FOCUS. Inevitably, a student will ask about making a choice between alignment of the front knee and the alignment of the pelvis. He or she will wonder whether to keep the front knee over the foot, thereby letting the opposite side of the pelvis turn inward, or whether to keep the pelvis pointing forward, thus letting the knee move over the foot.

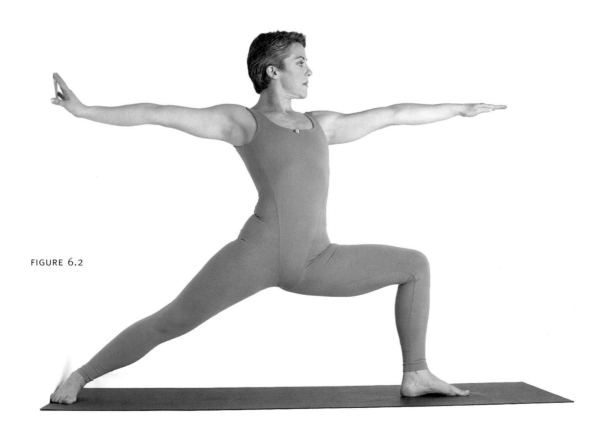

FIGURE 6.2

The more important of these two considerations is the alignment of the front knee. The knee joint is most stable when it is straight and does not bear weight; it is least stable when it is bent and bears weight. In this pose, the front knee is placed in an unstable position because it is both bent and bearing weight. Therefore, advise your student to focus on the alignment of the front leg to assure optimum protection of the knee. Of course, it is still important to try to maintain pelvic alignment, but not at the cost of the health of the front knee.

PRIMARY ADJUSTMENT. Try this simple technique to help your student experience the power of stretching through the back arm in Warrior II Pose. Stand by the student's back foot. After asking and receiving permission to touch him or her, firmly hold the student's fingertips with one of your hands and gently pull backward as the student moves into the bent knee position. Your touch should make it slightly more difficult for the student to bend the front knee, but not impossible. This experience will help the student to bring awareness to the back arm, as well as to the importance of finding a balance between stretching backward and moving forward.

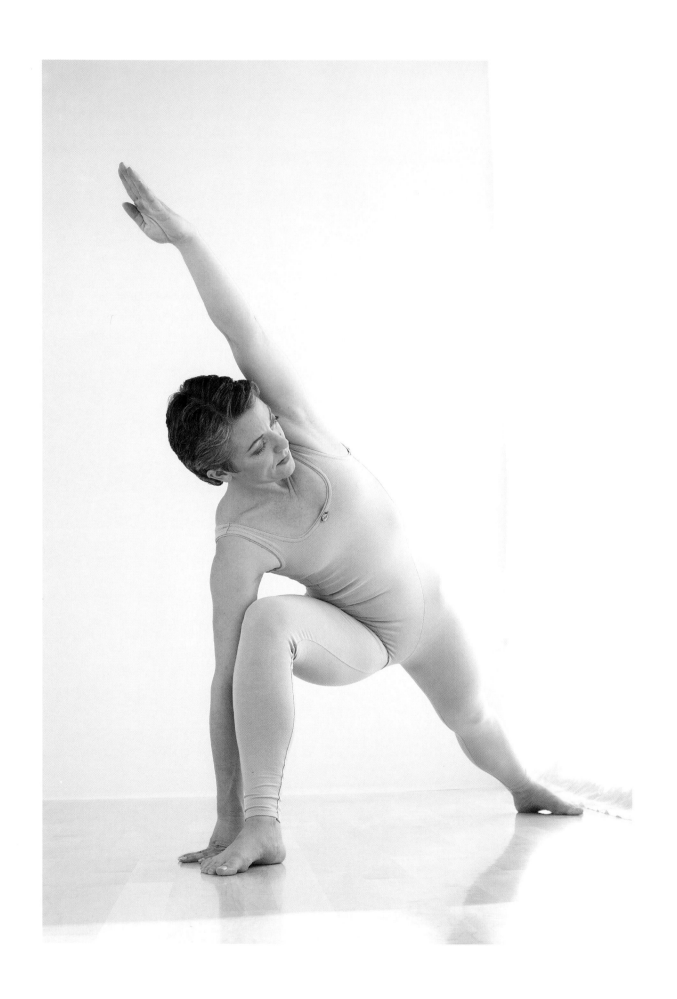

Extended Side-Angle Stretch Pose
Utthita Parsvakonasana

7

EXTENDED SIDE-ANGLE STRETCH POSE (Utthita Parsvakonasana) is one of the most beautiful of the standing asana. It requires openness in the hips and strength in the legs, as well as awareness in the upper body. The diagonal line created by the arm, torso, and leg symbolizes our connection from Earth to heaven and heaven to Earth.

This pose is particularly adaptable to students of all levels. It is physically challenging for the beginner and mentally challenging for the more experienced student. It provides a wonderful antidote to sitting all day in a chair with the legs close together.

SEQUENCING. This pose follows logically after Extended Triangle Pose (Figure 3.1) or Warrior II Pose (Figure 6.1). Occasionally, you can practice it before Extended Triangle Pose.

BENEFITS. Extended Side-Angle Stretch Pose creates flexibility in the hip joints, improves balance, stretches the inner thighs, strengthens the leg muscles, and opens the chest and shoulders.

CAUTIONS. Extended Side-Angle Stretch Pose is not recommended during the menstrual period or when your balance may be shaky, such as when you are recovering from the flu. If the latter is the case, then practice with your back to the wall for added support. Avoid this pose if your knees are swollen or painful, and after the sixth month of pregnancy. If you have diagnosed disc disease in your lower back, then practice this pose under the guidance of your yoga teacher.

The Essential Pose *(Figure 7.1)*

PROP: 1 nonskid mat

Spread your mat on a firm and level surface, and stand on it in Mountain Pose (Figure 1.1). Separate your feet about 4 to 4½ feet apart, lift your arms to the sides, and turn your feet to the right as for Extended Triangle Pose (Figure 3.1). Then bend your front knee as for Warrior II Pose (Figure 6.1).

Once your leg is in the shape of a carpenter's square, stretch your right arm and torso over the front leg, placing your right fingertips on the floor and to the outside of your right foot. At the same time, extend your left arm overhead and parallel to your left ear. As you move, breathe softly and keep your legs still. Be careful not to drop down farther by bending your front leg more and thus moving your knee past your foot.

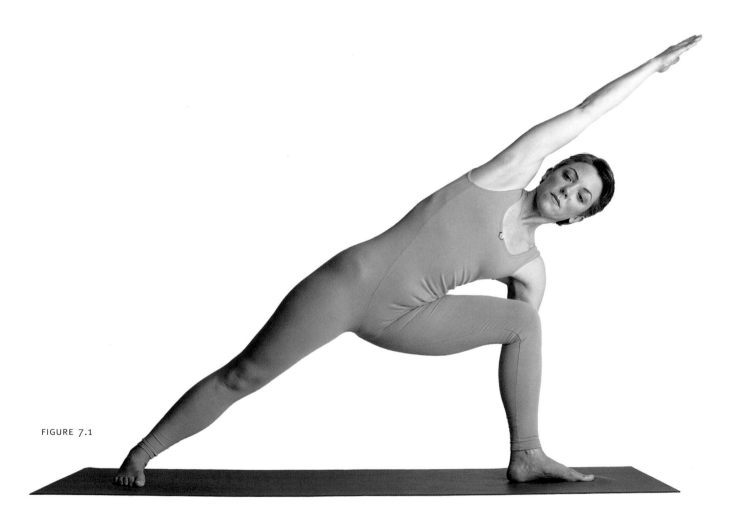

FIGURE 7.1

Turn your chest toward the ceiling. Hold Extended Side-Angle Stretch Pose for several breaths. To come up, inhale and turn your palm toward the ceiling and extend through that palm. This little trick will help you come up with a minimum of effort. Take a few breaths and practice the pose on the other side.

EXPLORATION. Extended Side-Angle Stretch Pose is a combination of skills learned in Extended Triangle Pose (Figure 3.1) and Warrior II Pose (Figure 6.1). The first part of the pose is exactly like Extended Triangle Pose and Warrior II Pose. When you are in those poses, you hold your body firm and stretch to the side, exactly as in Extended Side-Angle Stretch Pose

Remember, tip your pelvis to the right as you stretch to the right. It is like turning your steering wheel to the right when you want to turn your car in that direction. Your pelvis turns as a whole, as it did in Extended Triangle Pose: it tips fully to the right as it moves around your hip joints. Thus, as you come into Extended Side-Angle Stretch Pose, your tailbone is no longer pointing down, but pointing toward the heel of your back leg. This action creates a true diagonal line from your foot, through your torso, and out your fingertips.

Next, drop your right ribs down, toward the front thigh. This helps you feel the openness of the pose, not just the stretch. As paradoxical as it seems, sometimes a student can use the stretching sensations of a pose to avoid the openness. In Extended Side-Angle Stretch Pose, the emphasis is not on stretching the upper side of the trunk but rather on letting the lower side of the trunk drop and rest on the thigh. This creates a more receptive feeling in the belly and chest, even in the midst of such a strong active pose. Extended Side-Angle Stretch Pose is a perfect example of how each asana is a balance between being active and being receptive.

VARIATIONS

Props: 1 nonskid mat ✦ 1 block

EXTENDED SIDE-ANGLE STRETCH POSE WITH YOUR HAND ON A BLOCK *(Figure 7.2)*. This variation can be a boon to the beginning student, as well as an interesting learning tool for the more experienced one. Before beginning the pose, place a block behind your front foot. When you stretch out with your arm, place your fingertips on the block. You will have an easier time in the pose and the extra space will give you a better chance to work with the alignment of the hips and chest.

Try this variation if you are in the early stages of pregnancy, as well as during the postpartum period, to make your pose easier and more enjoyable.

EXTENDED SIDE-ANGLE STRETCH POSE WITH YOUR ARM SUPPORTED ON YOUR THIGH *(Figure 7.3)*. Practice this variation if you do not have a block or for variety. Once you have created the square with your legs, stretch out and, instead of placing your fingers on the block or the floor, place your forearm across your thigh and lean on it. You can use your thigh as the foundation from which to open your chest. Gently pressing back with your forearm can help you open your front hip.

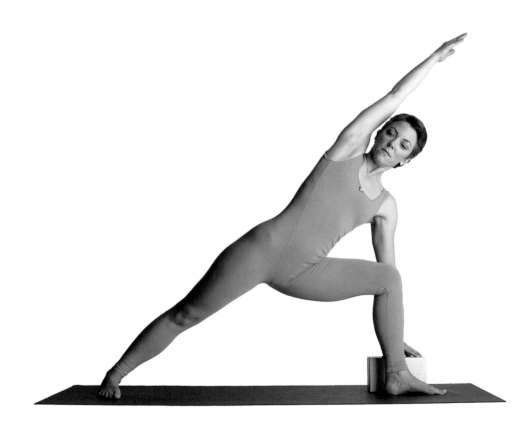

FIGURE 7.2

ESPECIALLY FOR TEACHERS

PRIMARY FOCUS. One of the difficult things about Extended Side-Angle Stretch Pose is the fact that the legs and the hip joints carry out opposite actions. As the student comes down into the pose, it is important that his or her knee stay over the right foot, with the hip strongly externally rotated, as previously discussed. But this action of external rotation is also important for the back knee. This double movement in opposite directions is what creates the basic openness of the pose. The foundation of counterbalancing movements from the legs allows for the opening of the chest toward heaven.

PRIMARY ADJUSTMENT. Take a moment to observe the shape of the student's front leg. The thigh should be square with the lower leg. This is determined not by the shape of the thigh, but by the relative position of the knee and the hip joints.

While the student is in the pose, visually draw a line from the center of his or her front hip joint toward the knee. That line should both be parallel to the floor and bisect the center of the knee joint. With this alignment, it may appear that the bottom of the student's thigh is lower than a squared position. But it is on the alignment of the joints, not the muscles, that achieves the relationship of evenness in the pose. Remember to encourage the student not to go past his or her physical ability to create the square, but to explore that limit and to work near it.

FIGURE 7.3

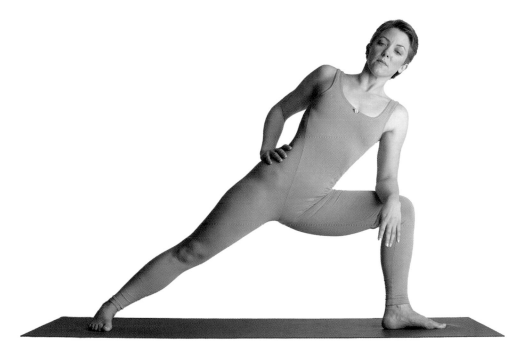

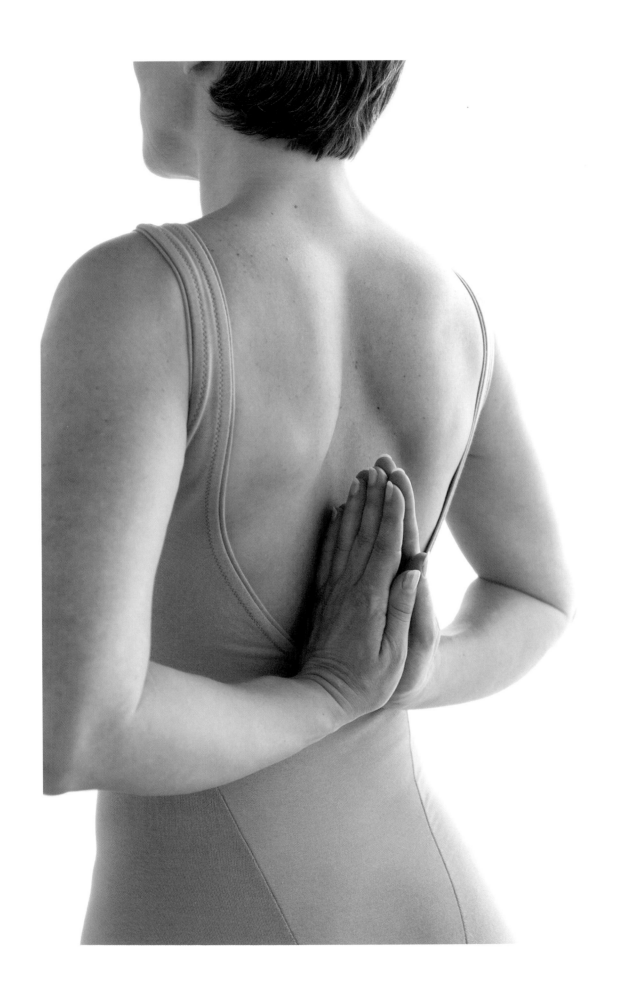

Side-Chest Stretch Pose
Parsvottanasana

8

SIDE-CHEST STRETCH POSE (Parsvottanasana) is a strong stretch for the arms and the legs. A student may find the arm position more difficult than he or she first expected. However, meeting the challenge is worth the effort. This pose creates flexibility in the wrists, a benefit that counters the negative effects of the wrist and arm positions that are held when working at the computer.

In addition to stretching the front of the chest and insides of the wrists, Side-Chest Stretch Pose is an intense stretch for the calves and the hamstrings. For the more experienced student who can bend forward with ease, the pose offers a pleasant compression on the organs of the lower abdomen.

SEQUENCING. Side-Chest Stretch Pose is usually practiced near the end of standing poses or after the more opening poses, such as Extended Triangle Pose (Figure 3.1) or Extended Side-Angle Stretch Pose (Figure 7.1).

BENEFITS. In addition to stretching the calves and hamstrings, Side-Chest Stretch Pose is one of the best asana for stretching the wrists and increasing shoulder mobility.

CAUTIONS. Side-Chest Stretch Pose is not recommended during the menstrual period or when your balance may be shaky, such as when you are recovering from the flu. Avoid it if your knees are swollen or painful when practicing the pose, if you have head congestion, or if you are uncomfortable with your head hanging down. If you are pregnant, you can continue this pose through the seventh month.

The Essential Pose *(Figure 8.1)*

PROP: 1 nonskid mat

Spread your mat on a firm and level surface, and stand on it in Mountain Pose (Figure 1.1). As you inhale, move your right arm away from the side of your body, about halfway between your leg and shoulder. As you exhale, bring your arm behind you and bend your elbow. Place the back of your right hand against your back, about midway between your shoulder blades. You may find it useful to wiggle your forearm up your back as you bring it into position. Keep your right arm in position as you repeat this procedure with your left arm. Remember to breathe.

Rotating from your shoulder joints, bring your elbows back. Continuing the rotation from your arms, press your palms together in Prayer Position, or Namaste, with your little fingers resting against your spine. You may find it helpful to bring your awareness to your shoulder blades as you come into this

FIGURE 8.1

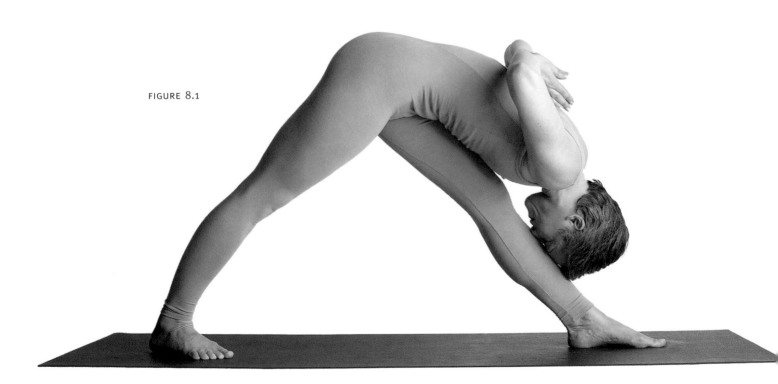

position. If you hold the shoulder blades close to the spine and slightly down toward the waist, then maintaining the hand position will be easier.

Separate your feet about 3½ feet apart. This distance is individual: the longer your legs, the wider the stance. However, do not position your legs at a distance that either compromises your stability or places a strong stretch on your inner knees once you have turned your feet. If either of these occurs, move your feet closer together. You can increase the distance between your feet when it is appropriate for you.

Classically, the pose is practiced with the forward heel (in this case, the right one) in an imaginary line with the middle arch of the back foot. However, you may feel more stable if your front foot is in line with the back heel. Exhale and pivot on your left heel, turning that foot in until your toes point toward the right. Inhale, and with an exhalation, turn your right foot out. If you do not feel stable or comfortable in this position, then try several placements of your front foot in relationship to your back foot, until you find the one that works best for you. Whichever one you choose, make sure that your back foot is turned well in and your front foot points away from you.

Turn your torso to the right, making sure that your hips are parallel with what is now the front of your mat. Inhale and keep your knees straight, pressing the back heel into the floor to facilitate stability and balance. As you exhale, slightly lean back, arch your spine, and bend forward from your hip joints. As you come down, lift and open your chest, and bring your torso over your front leg. If it is possible for you, bring your head toward your shin, but *not* at the expense of rounding your back.

Keep your breathing natural and easy throughout the next series of movements. With the torso down, swing it over the left leg *as you turn your feet to the left.* Stabilize the change of position by taking several breaths. Come up on an inhalation. Repeat the pose on the left side. After coming over your left leg, turn your feet forward *as you swing your torso* to the center. Inhale and come up.

Once up, strongly press your hands together, and then sweep them down and out to release them. You may enjoy stretching your wrists in the opposite direction. With an exhalation, step into Mountain Pose in readiness for the next pose.

EXPLORATION. Although the hands traditionally are placed in the front of the body, not the back, the joining of the palms is part of the Indian greeting that also includes bowing and saying "Namaste." The hand position is the physical acknowledgment of the joining of universal opposites to express an underlying oneness: left and right, night and day, matter and spirit, you and me, and finally all beings with the Divine. You express this understanding when you join your hands in Side-Chest Stretch Pose.

When in the pose, firmly press the bases of the fingers of both hands together. You may find that it is easier for the little-finger sides of your hands to have contact than the index finger or thumb sides. Keep the pressure even to afford a symmetrical stretch to the muscles on the fleshy side of the forearms, which can get tight from hours spent at the computer. Maintaining the awareness necessary to keep the pressure even is fundamental to this pose.

Another challenging aspect of this pose is keeping the elbows lifted and drawn back as you bend forward. It is so easy to let them drop. Think of your elbows as a focal point. With each exhalation, check within to sense the position of your elbows.

VARIATION

PROP: 1 nonskid mat

SIDE-CHEST STRETCH POSE, HALFWAY DOWN *(Figure 8.2)*. Another practice option is to come halfway down. This will help you keep your back long, as your leg muscles stretch. It is essential to keep your head down and face parallel to the floor as you lower and raise your torso to and from the halfway position. Lifting your head can feel uncomfortable for your neck.

Initially, you may find it almost impossible to join your palms behind your back. If so, practice with the arms folded and resting on the small of the back. Reverse the position of the arms when you practice the pose to the second side.

FIGURE 8.2

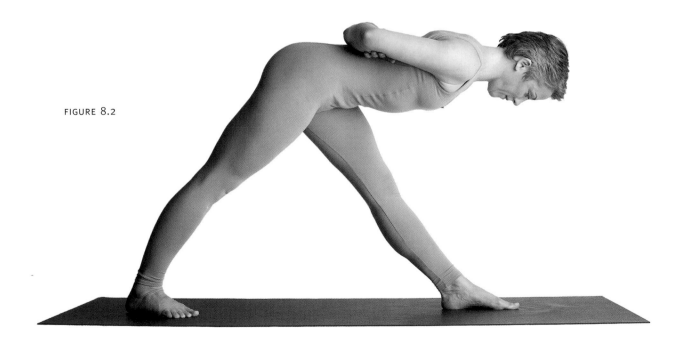

ESPECIALLY FOR TEACHERS

PRIMARY FOCUS. This is one of the more difficult standing poses, because of the equal involvement of the lower and upper body. A common problem is that a student's front foot tends to roll to the little-toe side, affecting her balance as she goes down. In part, this difficulty can be prevented if the student does two things. First, she should focus on firmly pressing the outer heel of the back foot down throughout the pose. Second, she should press the ball of the front foot down to avoid rolling out. The paradox is that at the same time, she needs to press out and back on the outside corner of the front upper thigh. Stability is created by the external rotation of the upper front thigh and the opposite movement at the foot.

Stability is the first rule of yoga practice. Without stability, all flexibility is just collapse. But when you move from a place of stability, you move from strength. You then have choice and power, whether it be in Side-Chest Stretch Pose or in your life.

PRIMARY ADJUSTMENT. To help your student create stability, give him feedback about the position of his pelvis. For example, when the pose is practiced to the right, the right side of the pelvis may move forward toward the right leg while the left side of the pelvis lags behind. This can contribute to instability.

After asking and receiving permission from him, gently touch your student around the upper rim of his pelvis, and help him to become aware of what an even pelvis feels like. You can do this by using your hands to demonstrate how the pelvis may be moving forward more on one side than the other. (In this pose, the front pelvis probably will be dropped a bit, but the pelvis should remain even from side to side.)

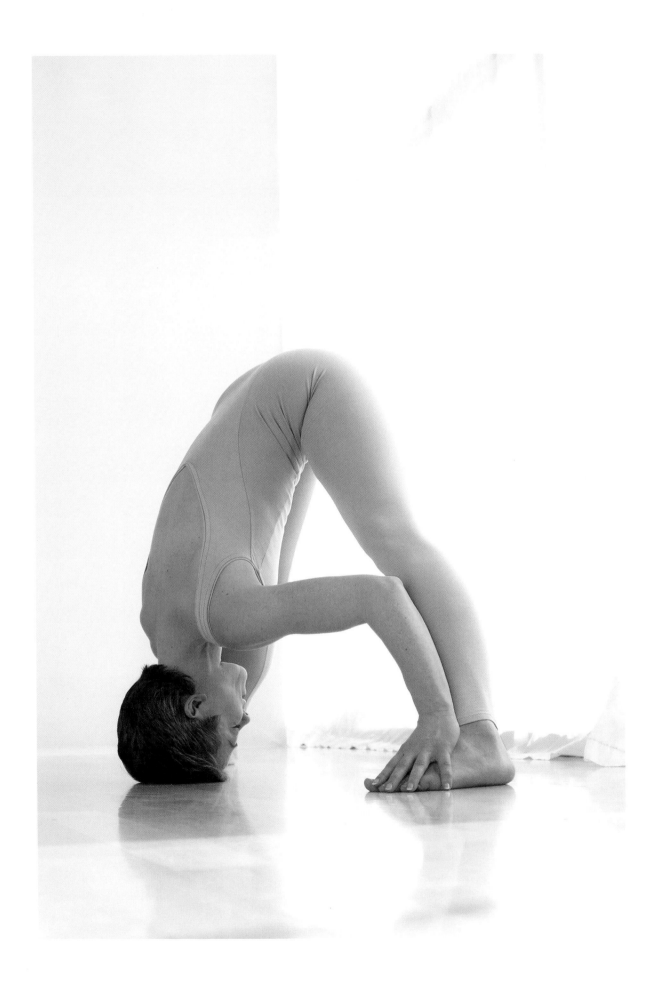

Wide-Leg Standing Forward Bend Pose

Prasarita Padottanasana

9

WIDE-LEG STANDING FORWARD BEND POSE (Prasarita Padottanasana) is a favorite among beginners and more experienced students alike. It is one of the *quieter* standing poses. This pose stretches the hamstrings, but more gently than poses in which the legs are closer together. It is sometimes taught by itself as a preparation for a practice centered on seated forward bends. Some teachers consider it a beginning inverted pose and a good preparation for more advanced ones, such as Supported Shoulderstand Pose (Figure 20.1).

SEQUENCING. You can include this pose at the end of your standing pose practice, as a rest between vigorous standing poses, as a preparation for a long practice of seated forward bends, or before or after Downward-Facing Dog Pose (Figure 10.1). In addition, Wide-Leg Standing Forward Bend Pose can be practiced before you begin inverted poses.

BENEFITS. This pose is a great stretch for the backs of the thighs and for the calves. It makes the hip joints more flexible and it strengthens the quadriceps.

CAUTIONS. Skip this pose if you are menstruating or have concerns about practicing with your head positioned below your heart. It is not recommended for those suffering from diagnosed disc disease, a detached retina, or glaucoma. Avoid this pose during the last month of pregnancy.

The Essential Pose *(Figure 9.1)*

1 nonskid mat

Spread your mat on a firm and level surface, and stand on it. Begin in Mountain Pose (Figure 1.1). Separate your legs about 4 to 4½ feet apart. Turn your toes slightly toward each other. Make sure that your knees are straight. Bend your elbows and place your hands on the outsides of your upper thighs, where your legs join your torso. Inhale and, with an exhalation, bend forward. Once you have come down, lightly place your hands on the outsides of your ankles. Breathe normally throughout the pose.

The most important practice point for this pose is to initiate and continue the forward bend from your hip joints and *not from your lower back.* In other words, your pelvis should tip forward so that your lower back is elongated and the arch in the lumbar spine retains its natural curve: it does not round up or out. You can accomplish this, in part, by keeping your abdominal muscles slightly active. If your lower back is in the right position, then your ribs will neither poke out nor be pulled in.

Check the photographs that accompany this text to make sure that you understand this movement. In addition, have someone watch as you practice and tell you about whether you are keeping your lower back concave.

FIGURE 9.1

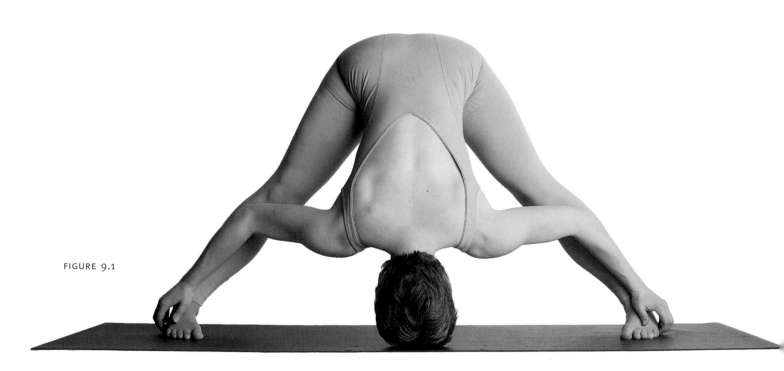

Hold this pose for five breaths. To come up, place your hands on your thighs just above your knees, and gently push down as you lift up. *To prevent dizziness, make sure that you take a big inhalation as you come up.*

EXPLORATION. Although Wide-Leg Standing Forward Bend Pose generally is considered an active stretching pose, it can become a resting one if practiced in the following way. After you have come forward, keep your breathing soft and allow your back to round slightly, thus letting go of the action of maintaining the lumbar curve.

There is an important distinction to be made here. Be sure to keep your back long *while* you are coming down. But once you are down, and if you do not require the use of a block, allow your back to round softly, inviting your belly to move inward and release. (To practice with a block, see the variation shown in Figure 9.2.) Then close your eyes and take several breaths, focusing on letting go not only of any tension in your hamstrings, but also of any tension in your mind. Practiced this way, this pose will help you to restore your equanimity.

VARIATIONS

PROPS: 1 nonskid mat   ✦   1 block

WIDE-LEG STANDING FORWARD BEND POSE WITH A BLOCK *(Figure 9.2)*. If bending forward from your hip joints and not rounding your lower back in the process seems like the impossible dream, then use the support of a block. This will help you to stretch the backs of your legs and to maintain the integrity of the lumbar curve, thus protecting your lower back.

Position the block directly under your shoulder joints so that your arms are perpendicular to the floor. Place the heels of your hands on the edge of the block with your fingers around the outside edges. (A beginning student may place the block too close to the body, thus increasing the likelihood that the back will round—exactly what the use of the block is designed to prevent.)

WIDE-LEG STANDING FORWARD BEND POSE WITH A SIDE TWIST *(Figure 9.3)*. When the essential pose (Figure 9.1) feels comfortable, try this delicious variation. Come forward with an exhalation, and then walk your hands toward your right leg, so that your breastbone is in line with your thigh. Place your left hand on the outside of your right ankle, and place your right hand on your side waist.

With the next natural exhalation, slightly contract your abdominal muscles, turn your belly to the right, and then release your belly once you are in the pose. Repeat the exhalation and rotation of your belly at least one more time. Imagine that you are turning not just your belly toward the right, but the belly organs as well. When you do this, your left hip will drop toward the floor. Hold for several breaths and then repeat to the left side by walking your hands across the floor in front of your body. Remember to keep your breath easy and to practice the abdominal contraction with an exhalation.

FIGURE 9.2

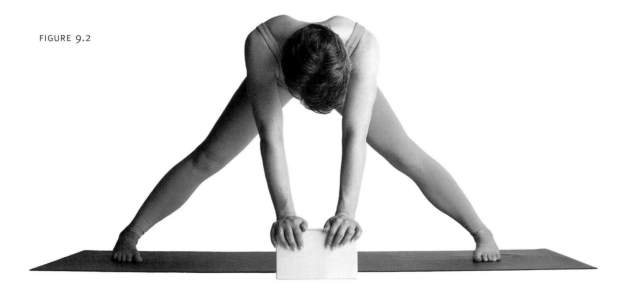

ESPECIALLY FOR TEACHERS

PRIMARY FOCUS. A student may not understand the importance of keeping a neutral lumbar spine when coming into and out of the forward bend. Ask your student to practice with one hand placed on the belly and the other on the lower back. Your student will be able to feel what happens when he or she bends forward and comes up. Generally, the experienced student arches too much, and the beginning student arches too little.

Another way for the student to experience a neutral spine and the work of the legs is to focus on the tailbone. When the student presses down at the tip of the tailbone as he or she bends forward or comes up, the contraction of the hamstring and buttock muscles is facilitated, thus creating less work for the erector muscles. When the student keeps the spine in a neutral position, his or her experience of the pose is that it is a movement that expresses equanimity.

PRIMARY ADJUSTMENT. Carefully watch the student from the front as he or she bends forward, to make sure that the hips are even. A student may practice with the pelvis slightly tilted to one side, thus putting more weight on one leg. He or she most likely will be unaware of doing this. It will, no doubt, feel a bit awkward for the student to shift the weight to even out the pelvis, but it is necessary if he or she is to prevent habitual overstretching of the back of one leg. And paying attention to how you act, whether in Wide-Leg Standing Forward Bend Pose or in other areas of your life, is what it means to practice—and live—yoga.

FIGURE 9.3

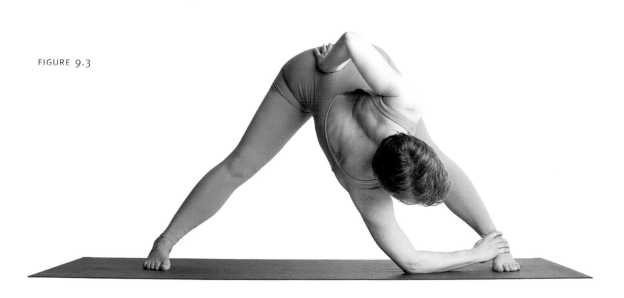

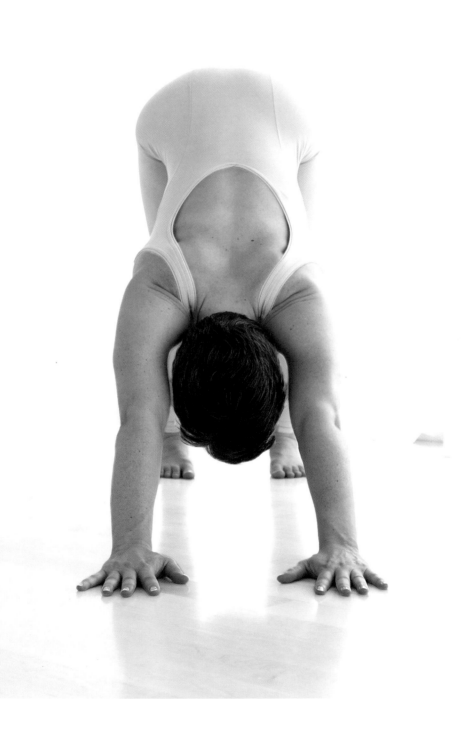

Downward-Facing Dog Pose

Adho Mukha Svanasana

10

IF YOGA STUDENTS VOTED for the most popular pose, Downward-Facing Dog Pose (Adho Mukha Svanasana) might very well win. Sometimes called Down Dog, it is often the first pose taught in classes and the one that students inevitably remember to practice on their own. That's great, because this pose is practically a mini yoga session all its own. My students love to say that a day isn't complete without Down Dog. I personally have practiced it in hotel rooms throughout the world, and once on a picnic table at a deserted campsite to relieve stiffness caused by hours of driving.

SEQUENCING. Downward-Facing Dog Pose is user friendly. You can start your practice with it; you can use it to prepare for forward bends and backbends; and you can practice it before and after most inversions.

BENEFITS. This is virtually a one-pose-cures-all asana. It stretches all the muscles in the backs of the calves and thighs, the shoulders, the belly, and the back. It strengthens the arms, relieves neck tension, and offers some of the benefits of inverted poses, including the stimulation of the abdominal organs and the relaxation of general tension. Down Dog can be used as a warm-up for jogging or other athletic pursuits.

CAUTIONS. Do not practice this pose if you have glaucoma or retinal problems, or if you suffer from a hiatal hernia. Stop practicing the full pose in the third trimester of pregnancy, choosing instead Half-Dog Pose at the Wall (Figure 10.2). You can practice at the wall if you have wrist problems, such as those caused by repetitive strain injury (RSI). Skip this pose during the menstrual period.

The Essential Pose *(Figure 10.1)*

PROP: 1 nonskid mat

Spread your mat on a firm and level surface, and stand on it in Mountain Pose (Figure 1.1). Kneel down, with your knees hip-width apart and your hands under your shoulders. Your fingers, especially the middle ones, should point straight ahead. Keep the bases of your index fingers in contact with the floor.

Inhale, and with an exhalation, draw your belly toward your spine, so that your abdomen is concave. With your next exhalation, lead from your belly and slowly lift your pelvis to form an inverted V with your body. Keep your arms and legs straight.

Inhale, and as you exhale, press your heels toward the floor and stretch backward. Although your heels may not reach the floor, continue to press them down. Make sure that your feet point straight ahead, so that your heels are not turning inward. Keep your breath moving slowly.

Slightly roll your arms inward, as you press your thumbs and index fingers into the floor. Move your shoulder blades toward your hands and your spine toward your pelvis. Think of moving your torso back and up, toward the legs, as if you were trying to stand up but your hands were glued to the floor. Imagine that your pelvis is lifting up and off your spine in a diagonal line toward the ceiling behind you. Keep your breathing steady. Slowly come down after five to ten breaths, and then repeat the pose. When you have finished, come down and rest in Child's Pose (Figure 28.1).

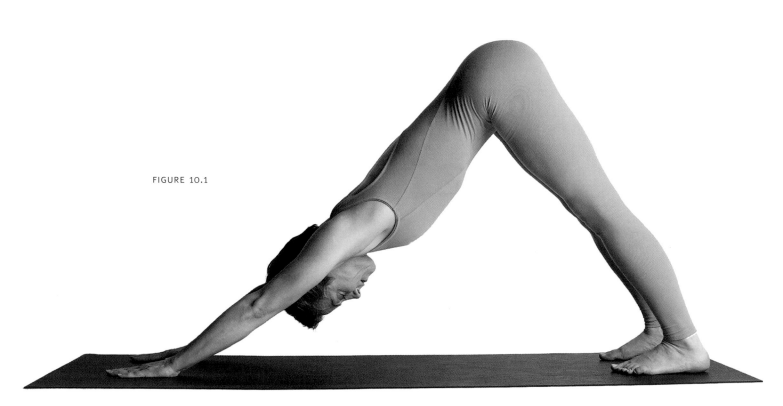

FIGURE 10.1

EXPLORATIONS. Practicing Down Dog with equanimity requires the balance of two opposites: pushing away with the arms and releasing the backs of the legs. In the Yoga Sutra, Patanjali names these two qualities *abhyasa* and *vairagya,* or "discipline" and "surrender." He states that spiritual practice is a combination of the two. They are beautifully expressed in Downward-Facing Dog Pose. If the leg muscles do not let go, then the pelvis will not tip, and the spine and shoulders will not elongate well. If the arms do not press back with strength, then the shoulders, spine, and legs cannot open properly. It is the balance and the blending, the harmony of *abhyasa* and *vairagya,* which creates the ultimate harmony in Down Dog—and in the rest of your life.

Another way to explore balancing opposites is to practice Downward-Facing Dog Pose with your heels turned out. In Western culture, many people have tight calves because they do not regularly squat. These very powerful muscles of propulsion and balance are also tightened by athletic endeavors, especially by jogging or running. In Dog Pose, turn your heels about halfway out. As you exhale, firmly press them down, without flattening the arches of your feet. Notice how much more stretch you feel in your calves. Hold for five to ten breaths, and come down with an exhalation. Repeat.

VARIATIONS

PROPS: 1 nonskid mat ✦ 1 wall

HALF-DOG POSE AT THE WALL *(Figure 10.2).* Stand at arm's length from the wall. Place your hands on the wall, at shoulder height, making sure that the bases of your fingers are in firm contact and your middle fingers point toward the ceiling. Inhale, and as you exhale, slowly walk your feet back, until your spine is parallel to the floor. Keep your feet hip-width apart and parallel, and your knees straight. Maintain the contact of your hands with the wall *and* push away from it, moving your shoulder blades toward your hands.

These movements are part of the gleno-humeral rhythm of shoulder joints that I describe in Warrior I Pose (Figure 5.1). If you find these movements difficult to understand while at the wall, then try them in a standing position. Step away from the wall. Lift your arms above your head, and then let your shoulder blades lift toward your ears. Now drop them back down. Try it again.

Once the movement feels familiar, try Half-Dog Pose at the Wall. Imagine that your spine is moving away from the wall, in the opposite direction from the shoulder blades. Then, with an exhalation, drop your shoulders and back down, to increase the stretch there and in your legs. Hold the pose for three to five slow breaths. To stand up, inhale and walk toward the wall. Repeat.

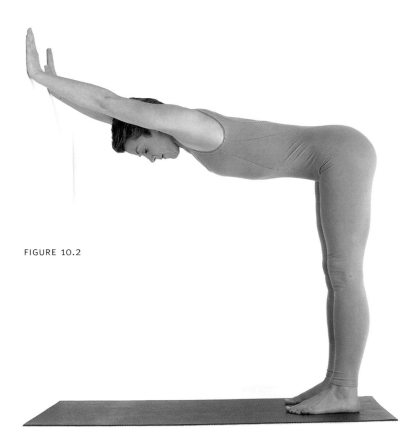

FIGURE 10.2

DOWNWARD-FACING DOG POSE WITH THE TOES OF ONE FOOT ON THE HEEL OF THE OTHER *(Figure 10.3)*. Here is another variation to stretch your lower legs and make your walking and running smoother. Come into Down Dog. Exhale, and place the space between the big toe and the second toe of your right foot on the lower part of the heel of your left foot. Firmly press down to increase the stretch in your lower left leg. Hold this pose for five to ten breaths, and repeat on the other side.

ESPECIALLY FOR TEACHERS

PRIMARY FOCUS. As a student becomes familiar with Downward-Facing Dog Pose, he or she may try to drop the chest farther and farther toward the floor. Unfortunately, this usually succeeds in overstretching the midback and understretching the lower back. Encourage your student to stretch evenly from shoulders to hips. One way to teach this is to remind the student not to push the front lower ribs out. The position of lower ribs in Down Dog should be like those in Mountain Pose (Figure 1.1): they lightly touch the skin. Remember, you want your student to focus on opening, not just on stretching to the maximum.

PRIMARY ADJUSTMENT. In the beginning, a student may limit himself or herself in Down Dog by placing the hands too close to the feet. Although there is no prescribed distance, make sure that there is room for the student's spine to elongate and the shoulders to open. The student may need to step the feet farther back. Suggest that your student experiment with the distance, so that he or she can avoid practicing what I call Puppy Pose, which looks almost like Standing Forward Bend Pose (Figure 11.1). Remember that Downward-Facing Dog Pose is not about dropping down, but rather about lifting up and off the spine and shoulder joints.

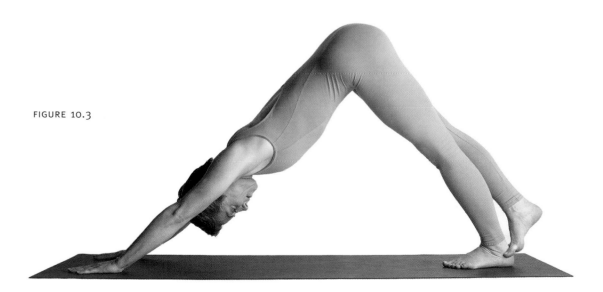

FIGURE 10.3

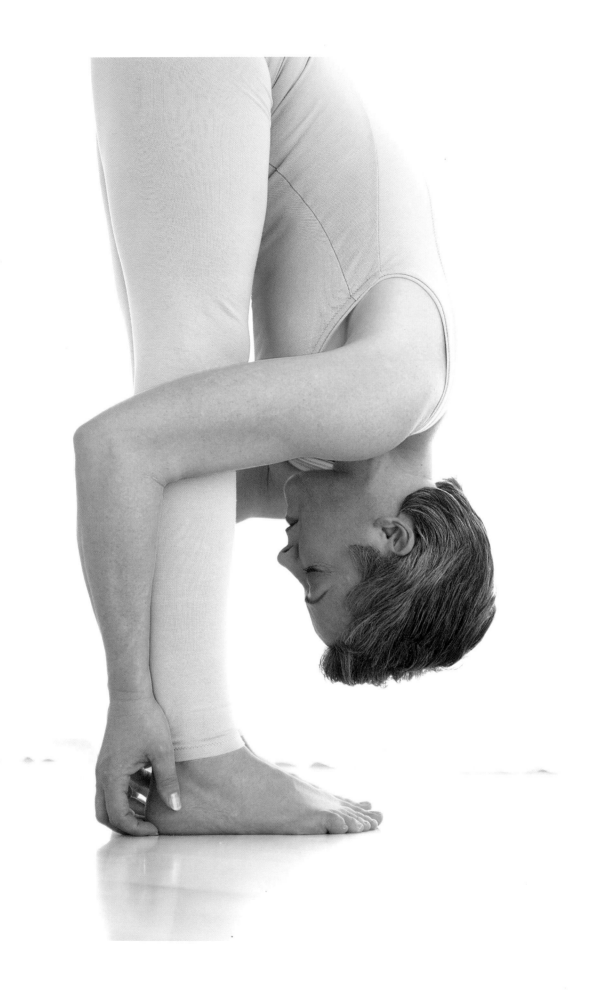

Standing Forward Bend Pose

Uttanasana

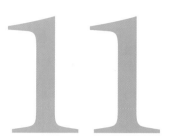

STANDING FORWARD BEND POSE (Uttanasana) is the simplest forward bend and is familiar to anyone who has done almost any form of stretching. It definitely stretches the hamstrings and lower back muscles, but must be done with awareness to decrease the possibility of strain in these areas.

SEQUENCING. Practice Standing Forward Bend Pose between the standing poses or at the beginning of a practice that focuses on stretching the hamstrings. On your nonskid mat, you can walk from Downward-Facing Dog Pose (Figure 10.1) into Standing Forward Bend Pose. In addition, practice it after sitting for hours.

BENEFITS. Standing Forward Bend Pose stretches the calves, hamstrings, lower back, and neck. In addition, it puts pleasant pressure on the abdominal organs. It is usually experienced as having a cooling effect on the brain and a quieting effect on the mind. As such, it will help you mentally unwind after a busy day.

CAUTIONS. Do not practice this pose if you have glaucoma or retinal problems, diagnosed disc disease, sciatica, a hiatal hernia, or a stuffy head or sinuses.

The Essential Pose *(Figure 11.1)*

PROP: 1 nonskid mat

Spread your mat on a firm and level surface, and stand on it in Mountain Pose (Figure 1.1), with your feet about 1 foot apart, your toes pointing straight ahead, and your knees straight.

Place your hands on your outer thighs, where they meet your torso. With an exhalation, bend forward from your hip joints, keeping your back long and stable—neither rounding nor arching—and the top of your head facing the opposite wall. Once down, lightly place your fingers on the floor, in line with your toes. Breathe softly as you carefully drop your head. Keep your weight forward toward the fronts of your feet. After five to ten breaths, come up with a strong inhalation and your back long, with a slight hollow in your lumbar spine. As you come to standing, bring your arms up and out to the sides in a big, arching movement, rather than lifted out in front of you. This movement will minimize strain on your lower back.

FIGURE 11.1

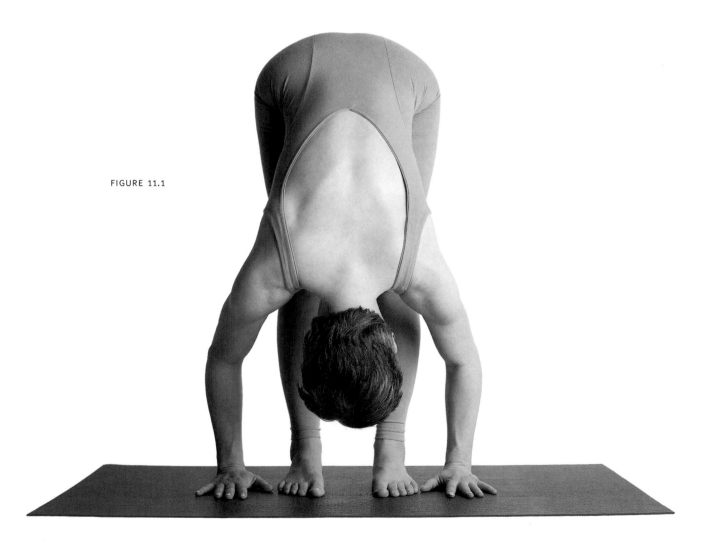

EXPLORATION. Moving from standing up to bending forward is an act of letting go, of coming inside, and of quieting down. As you bend forward, firmly draw your abdomen toward your spine with an exhalation. When in the pose, bring your attention to releasing not only the backs of your legs but also your neck and *especially* your belly. Keeping your abdomen concave and relaxed will facilitate deeper relaxation.

VARIATIONS

PROPS: 2 nonskid mats   ✦   1 block

STANDING FORWARD BEND POSE WITH YOUR HANDS ON A BLOCK *(Figure 11.2)*. Stand on your mat in Mountain Pose (Figure 1.1), with your feet about 1 foot apart, your toes pointing straight ahead, and your knees straight. Place your block between and slightly in front of your feet. When you come forward, the block should be directly under your shoulder joints, so that your arms are perpendicular to the floor and not reaching out in front of you.

Bend your elbows and place your hands on your outer thighs, where they join your torso. With an exhalation, bend forward from your hip joints, keeping your back long and stable, neither rounded nor arched. Now place the heels of your hands on the block, with your fingers around the outside edges. Keep your breath even, your elbows straight, and your lower back concave. After three to seven breaths, place your hands on your hips and come up with a deep inhalation.

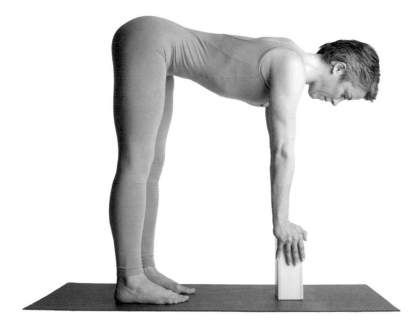

FIGURE 11.2

STANDING FORWARD BEND POSE WITH A ROLLED MAT UNDER YOUR TOES *(Figure 11.3)*. This variation will give an extra stretch to your calf muscles. Begin by folding the short end of your mat about 10 inches. Then fold that portion in half and firmly roll it. The sticky quality of the nonskid mat will help keep the roll in place. Stand with your feet about 1 foot apart, your toes pointing straight ahead, and your knees straight. Place the rolled portion of your mat under the front parts of your feet. Firmly press your heels into the floor to create stability.

Bending your elbows, place your hands on your outer thighs where they join your torso. With an exhalation, bend forward from your hip joints, keeping your back long and stable, neither rounded nor arched. Either use the block or place your fingers on the floor alongside your feet, so that the tips of your fingers are in line with the tips of your toes. After three to seven breaths, place yours hands on your hips and come up with a deep inhalation.

STANDING FORWARD BEND POSE WITH A ROLLED MAT UNDER YOUR HEELS *(Figure 11.4)*. This variation will give an extra stretch to your hamstring muscles. Fold and roll your mat as for Standing Forward Bend Pose with a Rolled Mat Under Your Toes. This time, however, place your rolled mat under your heels. Firmly press the balls of your feet into the floor to create stability. With your hands on your hips, come forward, placing your hands either on a block or on the floor. After three to seven breaths, place your hands on your hips and come up with a deep inhalation.

ESPECIALLY FOR TEACHERS

PROPS: 1 chair ✦ 1 nonskid mat
1 wall

PRIMARY FOCUS. Forward bends are often difficult because of tight hamstrings; this condition is caused, in part, by sitting a lot. Unfortunately, even physical exercise, such as jogging or working out, can tighten hamstrings. The only thing that does not tighten the hamstrings is actively stretching them in poses such as Standing Forward Bend Pose.

The primary focus in this pose is to make sure that the student is bending forward from the hip joints and the lumbar spine. Ask the student to get down on all fours, and tip the pelvis back and forth over the hip joints to get the feeling of what

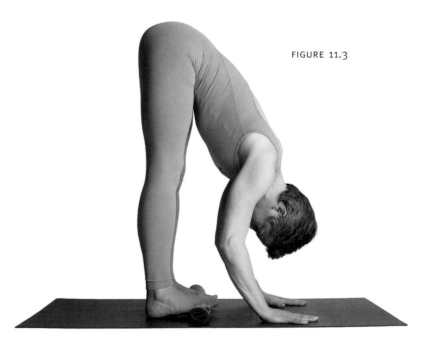

FIGURE 11.3

this is like. This movement is sometimes called Cat-Cow Pose or Pelvic Tilt Pose. Remember, it is done both ways: the tailbone points down and then up.

After your student has tried this movement on the floor, have him or her try Standing Forward Bend Pose, focusing on moving from the hip joints in a similar manner. If your student is particularly tight, then have him or her use a chair seat to support the hands when bending forward.

Another teaching aid is the wall. Have your student lean the back against a wall, with the feet spread about 1 foot apart and about 1 foot from the wall. As the student exhales, have him or her bend forward, moving the tailbone up the wall. When the tailbone stops moving is when the student is bending from the back and not the hip joints.

PRIMARY ADJUSTMENT. Practicing yoga poses is, in part, about becoming aware of habitual movement patterns. In Standing Forward Bend Pose, students often do three things. The first and most common tendency is to bend forward from the back and not the hip joints, which I have already discussed. The other two tendencies are to turn the feet out and to bend forward by pushing the legs back instead of keeping them perpendicular.

Make sure that your student has the feet placed with the toes pointing straight ahead. This means that if you were to draw lines between the second and third toes and a line between the anklebones, the lines would form right angles at the outsides and insides of the lower legs. A student may think that the feet are turning in when he or she tries this position. In fact, the feet are actually in neutral with respect to rotation.

Finally, watch from the side as the student bends forward. A student may push backward with the legs and pelvis as he or she does so. Pushing back can hyperextend the knee joints, which contributes to instability there. Suggest that your student keep the legs perpendicular to the floor as he or she bends.

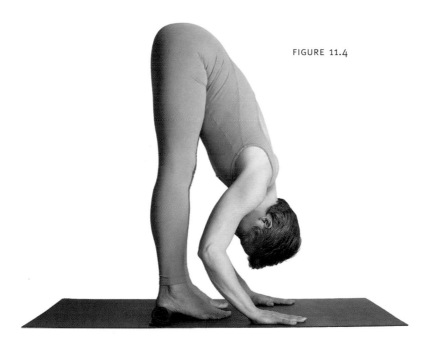

FIGURE 11.4

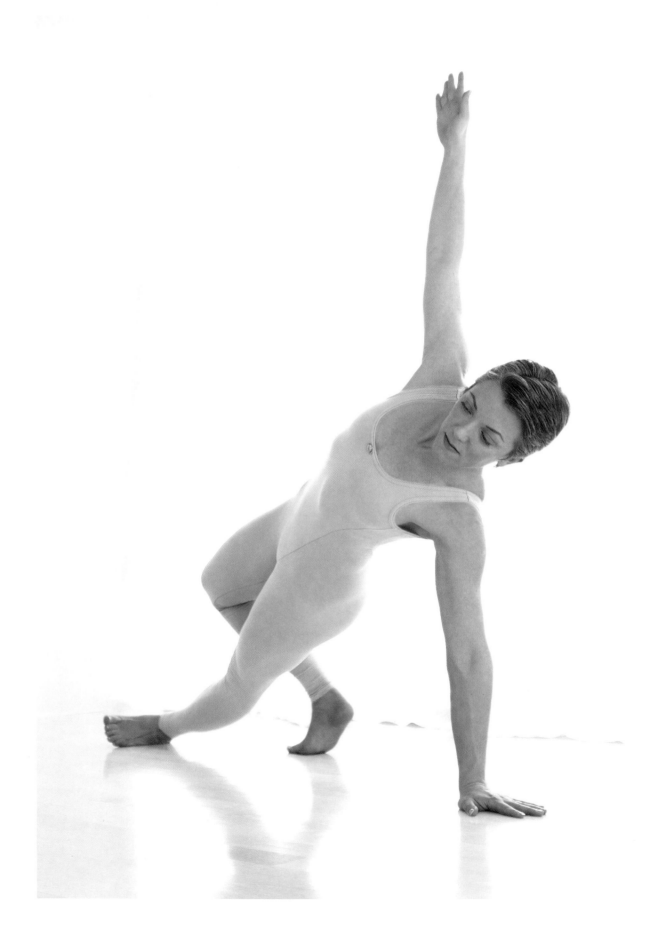

Up-Plank Pose and Down-Plank Pose

Chaturanga Dandasana

12

YOGA PRACTICE is well known for increasing flexibility. But a balanced yoga practice also includes poses that challenge the student to develop strength. Both strength and flexibility are necessary for a well-rounded practice *and* a balanced life.

Up-Plank Pose and Down-Plank Pose (Chaturanga Dandasana) will strengthen your arms and upper body. The first part of the pose is possible for almost everyone to try; the second requires much more strength. Both strengthen the triceps and the pectorals, as well as the abdominal muscles, which act as stabilizers.

SEQUENCING. Practice Up-Plank Pose and Down-Plank Pose just after Downward-Facing Dog Pose (Figure 10.1) or at the end of your standing poses, especially if you are focused on building strength. Experienced students can come from Downward-Facing Dog Pose to Up-Plank Pose and then to Down-Plank Pose as a flow sequence, which is called *vinyasa*. You can learn this flow by moving back and forth from Downward-Facing Dog Pose to Up-Plank Pose several times.

BENEFITS. Not only do these poses strengthen the muscles of the upper body and torso, but they also give you a boost of energy and confidence.

CAUTION. Do not practice this pose if you are suffering from a wrist injury, especially from repetitive strain injury (RSI). You can try Headstand Preparation Pose (Figure 13.1) instead.

The Essential Pose *(Figure 12.1 and Figure 12.2)*

PROP: 1 nonskid mat

Begin with Up-Plank Pose (Figure 12.1). Spread your mat on a firm and level surface, and get down on your hands and knees. Exhale and slowly stretch one leg back so that the knee is straight. With the next exhalation, place your other leg beside it. Your feet should be about 6 to 8 inches apart, and your toes curled under. Balance on your hands and your feet. Make sure that your body is in a straight line from your shoulders to your feet. Keep your breath fluid. Hold for three to five breaths, and come out by bending your knees and sitting back on the floor. Repeat this pose up to three times.

In Up-Plank Pose, a student often either lifts the hips too much or sags at the belly and lower back. For the first couple of times that you practice it, ask someone to observe your pose and tell you if you are in a straight line. As you practice, you will get a better sense of your body shape.

To practice Down-Plank Pose (Figure 12.2), begin by assuming Up-Plank Pose. With an exhalation, lower your body almost to the floor but do not allow it to touch the floor. *Chatur* means "four" and *anga* means "limb"; *danda* is translated as "staff" or "rod." In Down-Plank Pose, your body looks like a stick with four limbs. Hold Down-Plank Pose from three to five breaths and release. Lie on the floor to rest

FIGURE 12.1

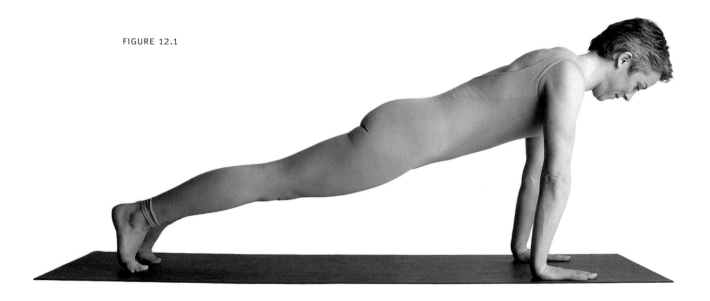

before repeating. As you become stronger, you can come out of the pose by pushing up to Up-Plank Pose.

EXPLORATION. There are two ways to practice Down-Plank Pose. One is to keep the elbows in close to the body as you descend, and the other is to let them go out to the sides. The first way is more strengthening for the triceps; the second way is more strengthening for the pectorals. Often men prefer the first way, women the second. Nevertheless, try both ways to round out your practice, especially if one seems impossible at first. If you try the second way, then you will probably enjoy the pose more if you put your hands slightly wider to start.

When you feel confident with this pose, you can then try to push up from Down-Plank Pose. Do this only if your arms and abdominal muscles are strong, and there is no feeling of strain in your back. Push up from Down-Plank Pose three times. Be sure to keep breathing as you work.

FIGURE 12.2

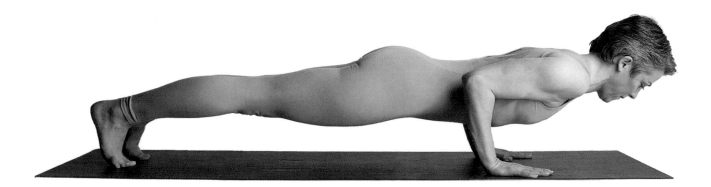

PROP: 1 nonskid mat

UP-PLANK POSE WITH ONE HAND UP *(Figure 12.3)*. When you are confident in Up-Plank Pose and Down-Plank Pose, try this variation. Practice Up-Plank Pose with your feet together. Then drop your heels toward the left, and lift your right hand up as you exhale to balance on your feet and your hand. Stretch your right hand up toward the ceiling. Be sure to keep your feet together and balance on the outside of your left foot, which is the little-toe side. Hold for three to five breaths, and come down by dropping your hand back to the Up-Plank Pose beginning position. Then practice the pose on the other side.

It might be difficult at first to keep from rolling backward in the pose. To prevent this, focus on rolling your pelvis forward as you open your chest in the opposite direction toward the ceiling. Remember to continue to breathe, even in the midst of the concentration that this variation requires.

FIGURE 12.3

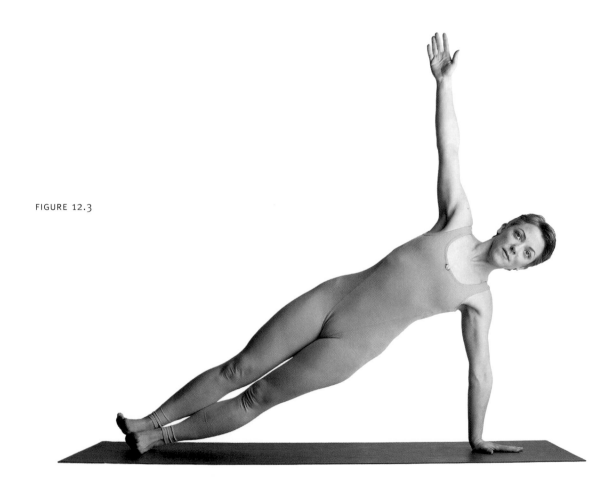

ESPECIALLY FOR TEACHERS

PROP: 1 wall

PRIMARY FOCUS. A student may think of these poses as supported only by the arms. It is important to remind the student to use the power of the legs when practicing Up-Plank Pose and Down-Plank Pose. The quadriceps can offer great support to the rest of the body if the student strongly presses back with the legs. Have the student try both Up-Plank Pose and Down-Plank Pose at the wall, with the student positioned so that his or her heels can press against the wall. This will help the student experience the powerful effect of using the legs.

PRIMARY ADJUSTMENT. When a student holds Up-Plank Pose, make sure that he or she does not sag in the middle of the body. Suggest that the student draw the muscles of the side abdomen toward the navel at the same time that he or she slightly presses the tailbone down. Of course, using the legs also helps; have the student press back through them, as described in "Primary Focus," and press them toward each other.

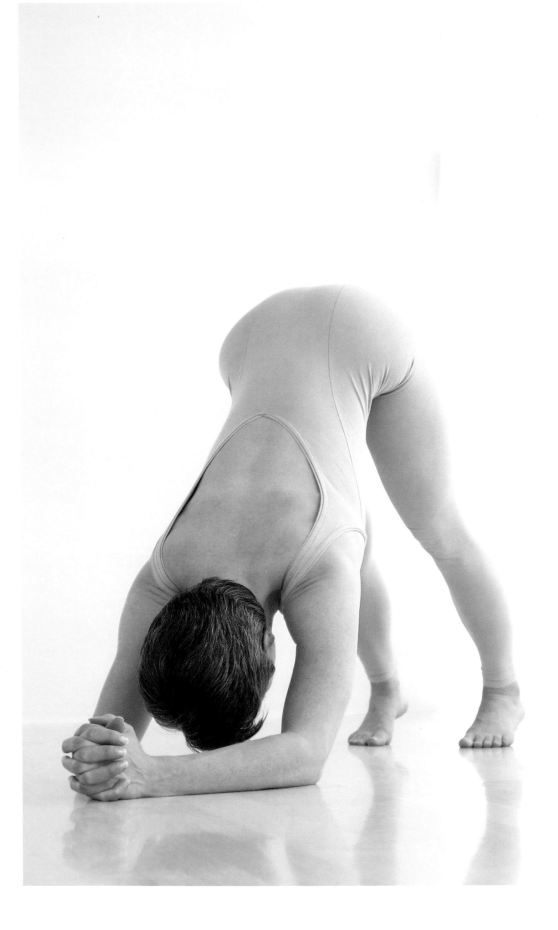

Headstand
Preparation Pose

Salamba Sirsasana

13

ONE OF THE POSES that is, in common imagination, most associated with the practice of yoga is Headstand Pose (Salamba Sirsasana). Not only will Headstand Preparation Pose (Salamba Sirsasana) prepare you for the full pose, but it is powerful and fulfilling on its own.

SEQUENCING. You can include Headstand Preparation Pose in practices that focus on building strength or shoulder flexibility. Practice Headstand Preparation Pose after standing poses or Downward-Facing Dog Pose (Figure 10.1).

BENEFITS. This pose offers one of the most effective combinations of strengthening and stretching the shoulders. It also increases flexibility of the upper back and hamstrings.

CAUTIONS. Do not practice Headstand Preparation Pose if you have glaucoma, retinal problems, or a hiatal hernia. Stop practicing Headstand Preparation Pose in the second trimester of pregnancy. During the menstrual period or if you have diagnosed hypertension, skip the variation called Headstand Preparation Pose with Your Feet on the Wall (Figure 13.4).

The Essential Pose *(Figure 13.1)*

PROP: 1 nonskid mat

Spread your mat on a firm and level surface. Begin on your hands and knees. Place your forearms on the floor so that your elbows are directly under your shoulder joints and your upper arm bones are perpendicular to the floor. Interlock your fingers and place them on the floor. Make sure that, although the roots of your fingers are touching, the palms remain apart and the wrists are slightly rounded. If you drew an imaginary line between your elbows, then it and your forearms and hands would form a triangle.

Turn your toes under. As you exhale, press back with your arms and lift your hips, so that your legs straighten and your weight is pressed onto your feet. You will probably feel a stretch in the backs of your legs and throughout your shoulder area. Your head should remain off the floor. Hold the stretch for five to ten breaths, and then come down on an exhalation.

Now practice on the other side. This time, the opposite thumb will be on the top and the other little finger will be on the floor. Notice how different the pose feels when you make this seemingly small change.

EXPLORATION. You can easily alter your experience of this pose by changing the position of your feet. To change the stretch in your legs and increase or decrease the stretch in your shoulders, move your feet farther back from your hands. To make the pose more difficult, move your feet closer to your hands. To make it easier, move your feet farther back and wider apart.

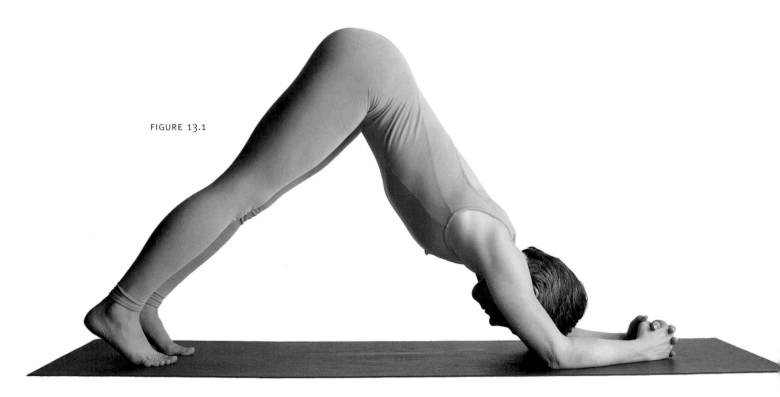

FIGURE 13.1

VARIATIONS

PROP: 1 nonskid mat

HEADSTAND PREPARATION POSE, MOVING BACKWARD AND FORWARD *(Figure 13.2 and Figure 13.3).* Assume Headstand Preparation Pose. Then inhale, and with an exhalation, move forward and backward over your hands. If possible, bring your body forward until it is parallel to the floor. Remember, exhale as you go forward and inhale as you lift back. Do not let your elbows move out to the sides. Repeat this process three to five times, and then sit back on your heels and rest for several breaths. Be sure to practice this pose again, this time with your fingers interlocked the opposite way.

FIGURE 13.2

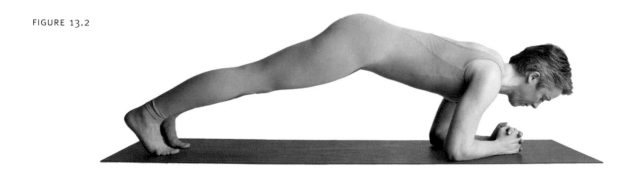

FIGURE 13.3

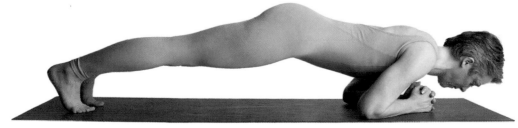

HEADSTAND PREPARATION POSE WITH YOUR FEET ON THE WALL *(Figure 13.4)*. This variation is sometimes called Half-Headstand. From the short end of your mat, fold it in half four times and place it near the wall. Your distance from the wall depends mainly on the length of your legs. Guess the distance the first time you try the pose, and then come down to adjust the mat if necessary.

Position your elbows and hands as in Headstand Preparation Pose. Turn your toes under and lift your hips. Lift from your shoulders so that your head is well off the floor. In fact, your head should never touch the floor in this variation. Carefully place the ball of first one foot and then the other on the wall, exhaling as you place each one. This position of the foot will give you some play in your ankle to adjust your distance from the wall. Eventually, you want your legs to be parallel to the floor.

Continue to lift from your shoulders by pressing your elbows down. Also lift from your thighs, which will help your spine to elongate. Keep your breath easy and flowing. Stay in the pose for five to ten breaths, and come down by bringing your feet down, one foot at a time, to the floor.

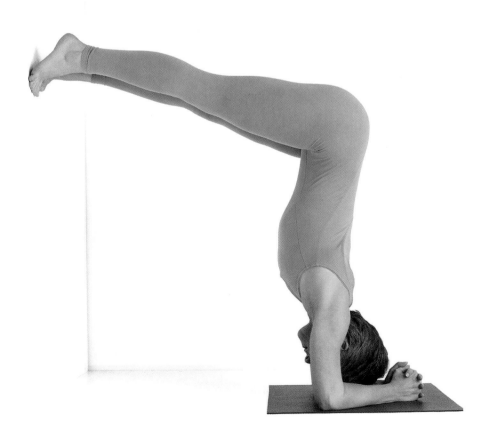

FIGURE 13.4

ESPECIALLY FOR TEACHERS

PRIMARY FOCUS. Although this pose is beneficial in and of itself, it can also begin to teach the student the proper alignment for full Headstand Pose. Make sure that your student learns Headstand Preparation Pose well from the beginning and is meticulous about the placement of the elbows and hands. As previously described, the elbows should be under the shoulders, and the upper arms should be perpendicular to the floor. The hands are fully interlocked, except for the little finger, which is released about 2/3 inch from the interlock.

When your student is in the pose, pay attention to his or her shoulders and thoracic spine. Some students use their shoulder flexibility and avoid their upper back tightness; others do the opposite. Suggest that your student even out the stretch between the shoulders and upper back to create a long line from the elbows to the outer hips joints. The midback should not be rounded or pressing in deeper than the diagonal line. If either of these happens, then make sure that your student understands the need to even out the stretch, and offer him or her specific instructions to do so.

PRIMARY ADJUSTMENT. To help your student get the feeling of lifting up and back in Headstand Preparation Pose, ask your student to assume the pose. Ask for and receive your student's permission to touch him or her for these adjustments. Stand behind your student, place your fingers on the outsides of the outer thighs, and pull diagonally up and back. Use enough force to help elongate the spine, without pulling so much that you lift his or her elbows off the floor.

For variation, stand facing your student's arms. Place the heel of your hand on his or her sacrum, and press diagonally up and back. Keep your fingers up, so that they do not touch his or her sacrum. Again, use only enough power to help him or her stretch the back and shoulders while keeping the elbows on the floor.

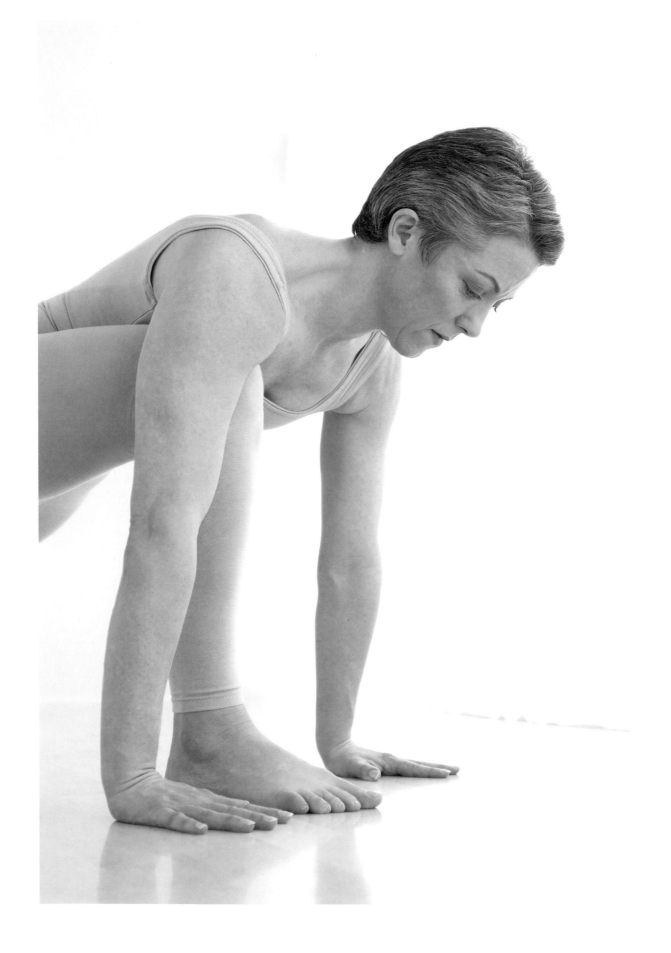

Lunge Pose
Anjaneyasana

14

LUNGE POSE (Anjaneyasana) is one of the few poses that beginners can safely use to stretch deeply the structures of the front thighs. If you spend a lot of time sitting at work or if you exercise frequently, then it is likely that your quadriceps muscles are tight. This tightness can contribute to lower back pain, as well as interfere with physical movement in sports and other activities. If possible, practice Lunge Pose every day to create more freedom in your walking and other movements.

SEQUENCING. This pose is a good preparation for back-bending poses. In addition, you can come into it directly from Downward-Facing Dog Pose (Figure 10.1).

BENEFITS. Lunge Pose stretches the short hip flexors and the quadriceps. When the knee is bent, the quadriceps receive an especially strong stretch.

CAUTIONS. Do not practice Lunge Pose if you are having knee pain or are recovering from a knee injury or knee surgery. Take care with the knee of your back leg. For comfort, you can place a folded face cloth under the kneecap. To avoid overstretching your inner knee, do not turn your back knee out (or drop your heel in).

The Essential Pose *(Figure 14.1)*

PROP: 1 nonskid mat

Spread your mat on a firm and level surface. Start from your hands and knees. Make sure that your knees are hip-width apart. Your hands should be under your shoulders. With an exhalation, lift your right foot and place it on the floor, between your hands, just a little to the right of center. Make sure that your right shin is perpendicular to the floor. This is the position of least strain for the ligaments of the knee.

As you place your right foot, straighten your back leg. Firmly push back through your left heel. Your left knee should be off the floor throughout the pose. Keep your breath soft. To increase the stretch, press down with your pelvis without letting your back knee bend. Hold for three to seven breaths. Come out by placing your right knee back on the floor and come onto all fours. Take a couple of breaths, and then practice the pose to the other side.

EXPLORATION. Once you are familiar with this pose, vary the stretch on the back thigh by turning that knee toward the other one. In other words, when the right leg is forward, turn the left knee toward the right. The left heel will drop outward by varying degrees, depending on where you want the stretch in the thigh. Experiment with different degrees of rotation to see which allows for the best stretch.

FIGURE 14.1

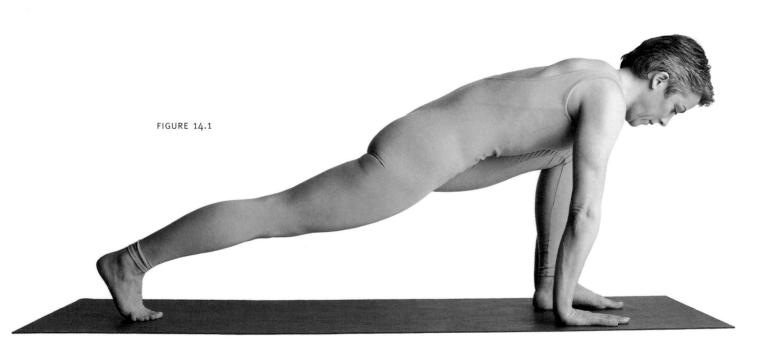

After you have stretched one side in the pose, get up and take a few steps around the room. Notice what a big difference the stretch makes to the sensation of freedom in your front hip joint. Practice this pose frequently to free your hips from the tightness caused by sitting or working out.

VARIATIONS

PROPS: 1 nonskid mat   ✦   1 face cloth

LUNGE POSE WITH YOUR BACK KNEE DOWN (*Figure 14.2*). Remember, move with an exhalation and keep your breathing normal during the pose. Come into Lunge Pose. To increase the stretch, slowly bend your knee and place it on the floor. You can place a folded face cloth under your left knee cap to give extra padding. Continue to press your pelvis forward; you may need to adjust the position of your front foot to keep your shin in a perpendicular position. Hold this stretch for three to five breaths, and then practice it on the other side.

FIGURE 14.2

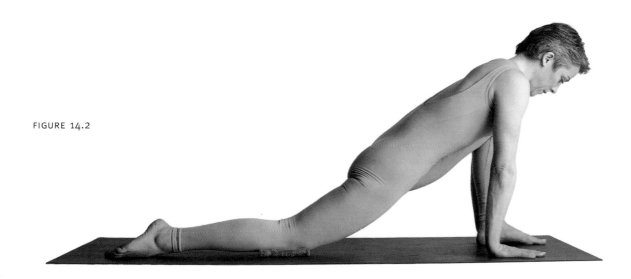

LUNGE POSE, HOLDING YOUR ANKLE *(Figure 14.3)*. This variation is very strong for the front of your back thigh. Try it only after Lunge Pose with Your Back Knee Down no longer feels so impossible to practice.

Practice this variation in two stages. To begin, come into Lunge Pose with your right foot forward. To increase the stretch, slowly bend your left knee and place it on the floor. Once it is comfortably there, bend your left knee and bring your left foot toward your hips. Do not lift your pelvis when you do this last action: keep your pelvis pressing down. Hold this variation for three to five breaths, and then practice it to the other side.

If you have tried stage one and want a deeper stretch, then drop your knee, reach back with your left hand and take hold of your left ankle, and pull your heel forward even more. Make sure that you do not lift your pelvis as you do. If your pelvis lifts, then practice Lunge Pose with Your Back Knee Down instead. This particular variation is undeniably a very strong stretch, so keep breathing. After three to five breaths, come out of the pose, and repeat it to the other side. After this variation, walking will feel like a new adventure.

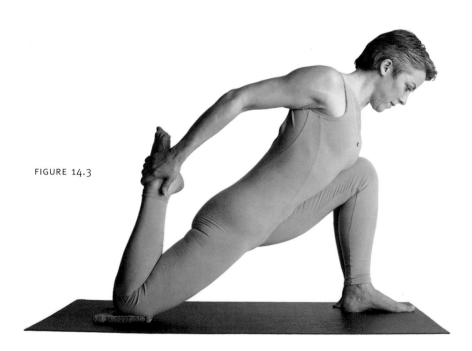

FIGURE 14.3

ESPECIALLY FOR TEACHERS

PRIMARY FOCUS. The knee joint is a vulnerable one, in part because it lacks strong muscular support. Therefore, it is important to make sure that your student keeps the front leg in healthful alignment during this pose. Double check to see that your student's shin is perpendicular to the floor. This means that there is no bend at the ankle. To the student, the knee may look vertical, but often there is a slight movement of the knee forward as he or she deepens the pose. Keeping the shin in this position will minimize stress to the inner and outer ligaments of the knee.

PRIMARY ADJUSTMENT. Although practicing this pose with the back knee down and heel drawn upward is a powerful stretch for the quadriceps, it can be uncomfortable for some students. The back kneecap may be sensitive to having weight placed on it. Suggest that your student place padding under the back knee. Additionally, make sure that your student has placed the weight of the leg above the kneecap and not directly on it. It may help to suggest that he or she move the front foot slightly forward to allow weight to rest above the back kneecap.

One of the most important things that yoga practice teaches is the difference between pain that must be experienced and that which can be avoided. The pain of pressing directly down on the back kneecap in this pose is a pain that definitely can be avoided by adding padding and changing the position of the back leg. However, the discomfort of the stretch in the back leg quadricep cannot be avoided if you are to stretch. Learning the difference between these two kinds of pain is the beginning of wisdom in practice.

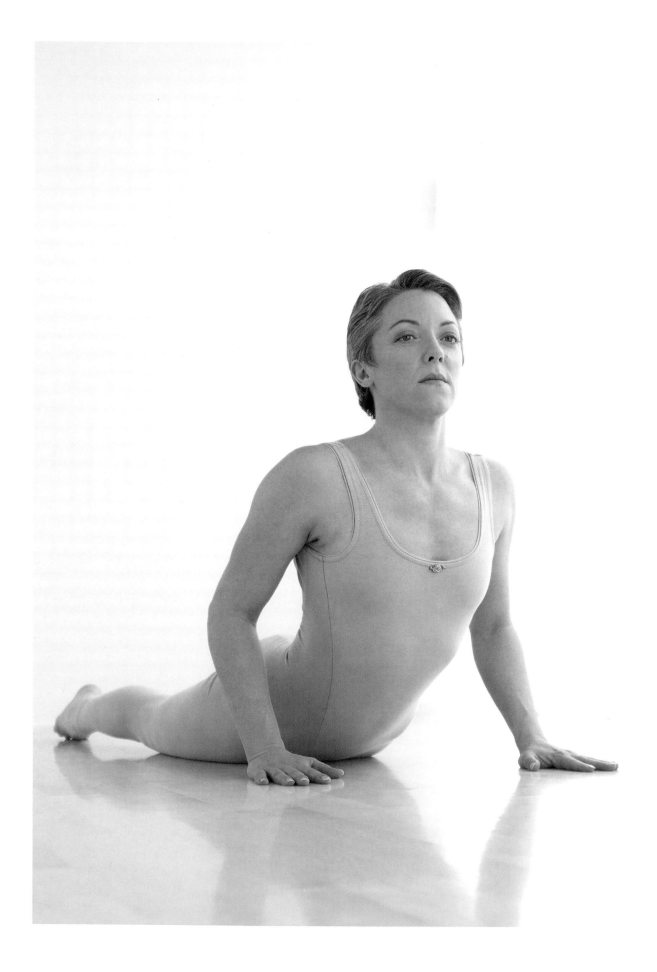

Cobra Pose
Bhujangasana

15

ONE AFTERNOON during my first trip to India, I was awakened from a nap by the sounds of a snake charmer playing his flute just below my hotel balcony. So gracefully and sinuously did his cobra lift up and sway out of the round basket that I was entranced and threw the expected coins down to a smiling snake charmer. Since that day, I have enjoyed practicing Cobra Pose (Bhujangasana) with the image of that snake in my mind.

SEQUENCING. Cobra Pose is usually practiced as the first backbend in a backbend series.

BENEFITS. Cobra Pose strengthens the long muscles of the back and those between the shoulder blades, and contributes to the improvement of erect posture. It stretches the abdomen and chest, and increases flexibility in the thoracic and lumbar spine. The thoracic area often stiffens with age, which is due, in part, to poor posture, especially when sitting. Cobra Pose is a great antidote to lots of sitting. Students who suffer from lower back pain and those with diagnosed disc disease find that Cobra Pose strengthens and relieves the back.

CAUTIONS. If you are pregnant, then do not practice this pose after the first trimester. Nursing mothers may find it uncomfortable. Seek the advice of an experienced yoga teacher if you have diagnosed disc disease, spondylolysis, or spondylolistheses.

The Essential Pose *(Figure 15.1)*

PROPS: 1 nonskid mat   ✦   1 blanket

Spread your mat on a firm and level surface. For comfort, fold a blanket and place it on the mat. Lie on the blanket. Lift one leg a few inches off the floor, and stretch it backward before setting it down on the mat. Repeat this action with your other leg. Your belly should feel long and in contact with the floor. Your legs are now slightly farther than hip-width apart.

Place your palms under your shoulders so that the tips of your middle fingers rest directly under your shoulder joints. Hold your elbows against your body, and draw your shoulder blades toward your waist and slightly toward each other.

Inhale, and with an exhalation, press down with your palms and slowly lift off the floor. It is *important* that your chin stay down and the top of your head face the opposite wall. This will keep your neck long and help you avoid crunching your neck in the pose. Let your gaze stay soft and rest on your lower lids.

It is equally important that you lift *and* keep your navel on the floor. Remember, a cobra has no arms. Control your lifting with your back muscles. Your arms are only *to help*. Imagine that the bend is coming from your midback. Stay in the pose for three to five breaths and come down. After a brief rest, try the pose again.

FIGURE 15.1

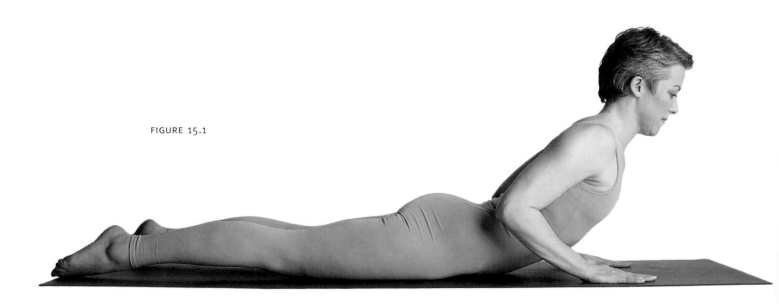

EXPLORATION. Cobra Pose aids in the flexibility of the upper back. It also stretches the front of the body, especially the belly. When you practice this pose, pay special attention to softening your belly and allowing it to stretch forward and upward toward your breastbone. One way that you can do this is to keep your legs firmly planted on the floor, gently pressing them down. It is this downward pressure that helps to create the upward lift of the pose.

VARIATIONS

PROP: 1 nonskid mat

COBRA POSE WITH YOUR ARMS STRETCHED TO THE SIDES *(Figure 15.2)*. Position your torso and legs for Cobra Pose. Place your arms out to the sides, palms down, so that you are in a T shape. Draw your shoulder blades down toward your waist and slightly inward toward each other. Inhale, and with an exhalation, begin to lift off the floor. Lift from your shoulders and make sure that your hands go no higher than your shoulders. Remember to keep your chin down and the top of your head facing the opposite wall. Hold the pose for three to five breaths and come down slowly. After a couple of resting breaths, repeat the pose.

FIGURE 15.2

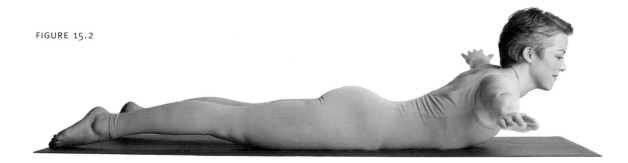

Cobra Pose with Your Arms Stretched Backward (*Figure 15.3*). Position your torso and legs for Cobra Pose. Place your arms along your sides with your palms facing your body and your thumbs turned toward the floor. Remember to draw your shoulder blades down toward your waist and slightly inward toward each other. Inhale, and with an exhalation, reach back with your arms, and lift them and your torso a few inches off the floor. Keep your chin down and the top of your head facing the opposite wall. Hold the pose for three to five breaths and slowly come down. Repeat the pose after a couple of resting breaths.

Cobra Pose with Your Hands Clasped Behind Your Back (*Figure 15.4*). Position your torso and legs for Cobra Pose. Reach your hands behind you, and interlock your fingers so that your palms face your head and are gently apart (as for Headstand Preparation Pose, Figure 13.1). Square your wrists. As you lift off the floor, reach backward with your arms *as if* you intended to hook your hands over your heels. Keep your chin down and the top of your head facing the opposite wall.

After a few restful breaths, repeat the pose. This time, reverse the interlock of your fingers so that your other thumb is on top and your fingers are shifted one space over. You'll know that you are getting this second position because at first it will feel unusual for your hands.

FIGURE 15.3

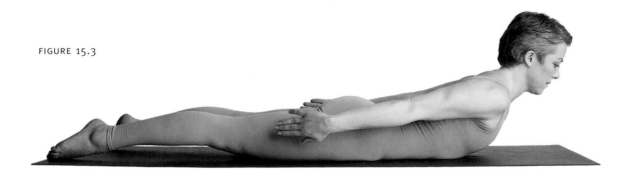

ESPECIALLY FOR TEACHERS

PRIMARY FOCUS. Almost without exception, students attempt to lift their heads first and arch their necks back as they begin this pose. This is not recommended for two reasons. First, the cervical spine and the lumbar spine are sympathetic curves. This means that they tend to move at the same time. If your student strongly arches his or her neck in Cobra Pose, then chances are that he or she will arch strongly from her lower back as well. However, the pose is designed specifically to create flexibility in the midback. Make sure that your student focuses his or her arch in this area and not in the neck and the lower back.

Second, initiating movement with the head and arching the neck is not a good idea because this brings the inner focus of the pose outward. A practitioner's focus tends to follow the direction of the eyes. When the student looks up, the focus follows. But when the student's head is dropped slightly and the gaze rests on the lower lids, he or she is more likely to remain relaxed and easy in the pose, with the focus inwardly directed.

PRIMARY ADJUSTMENT. Observe your student's sacrum in Cobra Pose. The sacrum is the convex curved bone that is part of the spine, and is located below the waist and just above the tailbone. Suggest that your student use this bone as the anchoring focus as he or she lifts. One image that facilitates healthful movement of the sacrum in Cobra Pose is to imagine that the top of the sacrum is being sucked down into the pelvis.

On the one hand, when your student imagines this movement, he or she facilitates the natural movement that occurs between the lumbar spine and the sacrum in healthful back bending. On the other hand, if your student were to tuck the tailbone in the pose, then he or she would interfere with this natural movement, which is called nutation. Tucking can cause lower back discomfort and should be avoided.

FIGURE 15.4

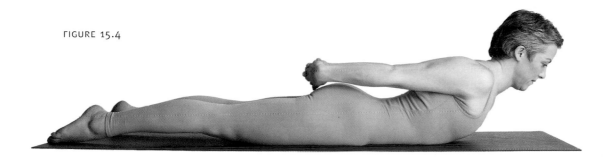

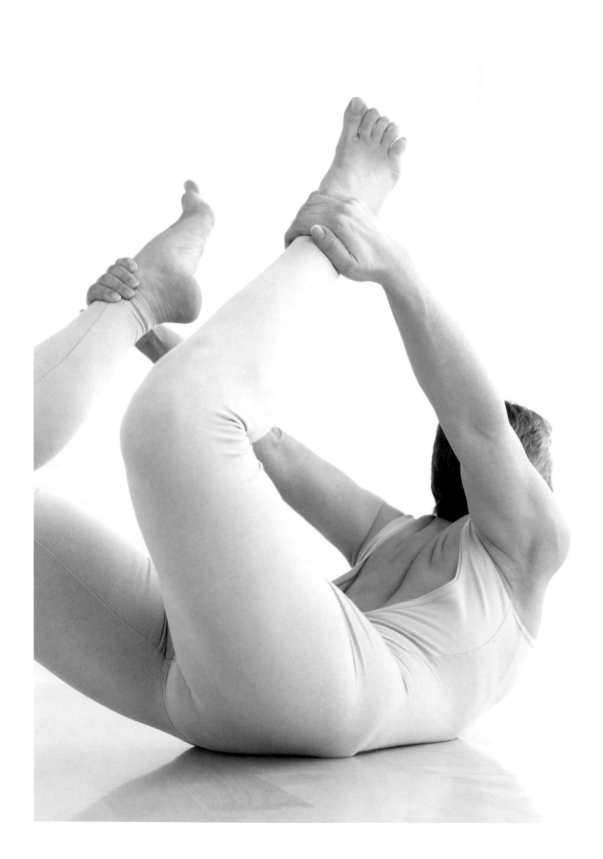

Bow Pose
Dhanurasana

16

ONE OF THE MOST RECOGNIZABLE ASANA, Bow Pose (Dhanurasana) is sometimes used in other forms of stretching. For example, my daughter practiced it in her gymnastics class, where it was called The Basket. Bow Pose is a backbend that beginners like, because it rarely bothers the lower back. It requires flexibility, not only in the shoulders, but also in the fronts of the thighs. It is energizing and helps to combat the effects of habitual sitting.

SEQUENCING. Practice Bow Pose after Cobra Pose (Figure 15.1) as part of a back bending series.

BENEFITS. Bow Pose strengthens all the muscles of the back and thus contributes to an erect posture. It stretches the abdominal and chest muscles and the fronts of the shoulder joints, and it increases flexibility in the thoracic and lumbar spine. Students who suffer from lower back pain and those with diagnosed disc disease find that Bow Pose strengthens and relieves the back. Finally, this pose is a great antidote to too much time spent sitting.

CAUTIONS. If you are pregnant, do not practice this pose after the first trimester. Nursing mothers may find it uncomfortable. Seek the advice of an experienced yoga teacher if you have diagnosed disc disease, spondylolysis, or spondylolistheses.

The Essential Pose *(Figure 16.1)*

PROPS: 1 nonskid mat   ✦   1 blanket

Spread your mat on a firm and level surface. Fold one blanket in quarters, so that it is approximately 2 feet long and 18 inches wide. Lie on your belly on your folded blanket. Take a moment to make sure that your belly and pubic bone are comfortable on your props. Lift one leg a few inches off the floor, and stretch it backward before setting it back down on the mat. Repeat this action with your other leg. Your belly should feel long and in contact with the floor. Your legs are now slightly farther than hip-width apart.

With an exhalation, bend one knee and catch the corresponding ankle with your hand. Then do this with the other leg. Make sure that your lower abdomen and upper thighs press down. If they do not, then practice Lunge Pose (Figure 14.1) until your front thighs are more flexible. Flexibility in your front thighs may help prevent lower back pain in the pose.

After you have grasped your ankles, inhale, and with an exhalation, lift your knees and shoulders straight up and off your blanket. Rest on your abdomen, just above the navel. Take three to five breaths and then slowly come down. Release your hands and straighten your legs. Rest for several breaths before you repeat the pose.

FIGURE 16.1

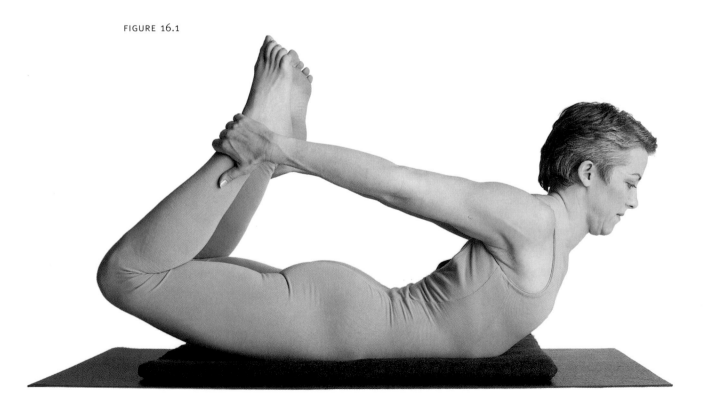

EXPLORATION. To enhance your sense of lifting up in this pose, focus on the top of your sacrum. Press down here to lift up everywhere else. Imagine a large boulder in a stream with the water flowing around it. Let your sacrum be like that stable boulder; let your arms and legs be like the water. Be sure to breathe as you incorporate this image into your practice of the pose. (When you focus intently, you may tend to hold your breath.

VARIATIONS

PROPS: 1 nonskid mat   ✦   3 blankets

BOW POSE WITH YOUR HANDS TURNED OUTWARD *(Figure 16.2) If you feel discomfort in your elbows, then do not practice this variation.* Position your props and your torso and legs as for Bow Pose. This variation calls for a different hand position. Make sure that you understand which way the hands turn in this variation, because it can be confusing. With an exhalation, bend one knee and reach your hand back toward the corresponding ankle. This time, turn your arm *out* so that your palm faces outward and your thumb points up, and take hold of your inner ankle. The last thing to check is that your shoulders and chest are opening as you practice these movements. Take care, because it is possible to turn your arm inward and still keep your palm outward and thumb up. This last action, which would collapse the shoulder, is *not* what I am suggesting.

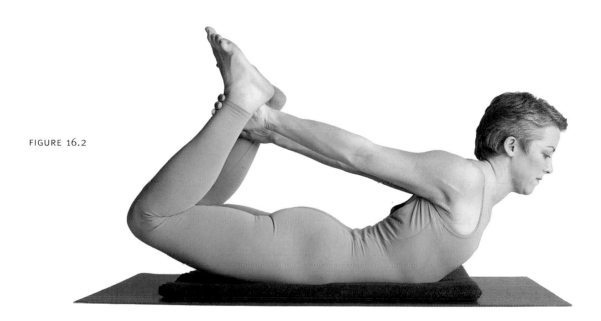

FIGURE 16.2

Once you are holding your ankle in this new hand position, then exhale and take hold of the other leg. Make sure that your lower abdomen and upper thigh areas are pressing into the floor. If this is not happening, then practice Lunge Pose (Figure 14.1) until your front thighs are a little more flexible. Front thigh flexibility may help prevent lower back pain in the pose.

After you have grasped your ankles, inhale, and with an exhalation, lift your knees and shoulders straight up and off your blanket. Rest on your abdomen, just above the navel. It is likely that you will feel a strong stretch in the pectoralis muscles. Take three to five breaths and come down slowly. Release your hands and straighten your knees. Take several restful breaths before you repeat the variation.

BOW POSE WITH YOUR HIPS ON BLANKETS *(Figure 16.3)*. Fold all three blankets into a rectangular shape that measures approximately 2 feet by 18 inches. Stack them so that the longest, firmest, and smoothest edges are on the same side. Lie on your belly on the blanket stack, so that your hipbones are just on those edges of the blanket stack and your knees are in firm contact with the floor.

Bend your knees and reach back to hold your ankles. With an exhalation, strongly press back on your legs, press down on your knees, and draw your chest up into an arch. Hold the pose for several breaths, making sure that your knees remain on the floor. Come down with an exhalation, and rest before practicing this variation again.

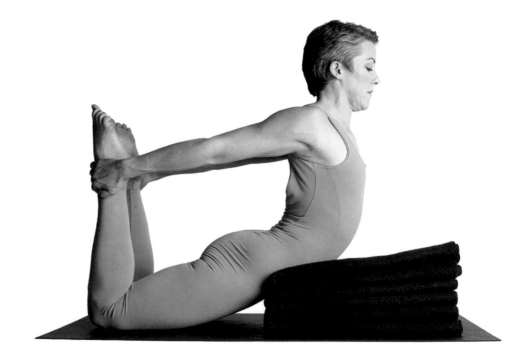

FIGURE 16.3

ESPECIALLY FOR TEACHERS

PRIMARY FOCUS. One way to help your student enjoy this pose is to remind him or her to lift *up* and not just backward in Bow Pose. Describe how the knees and the shoulders should move up in a straight line, so that they are equidistant from the floor. These instructions will help your student equalize the backbend and avoid overarching either the cervical spine or the lumbar spine. Remember, it is the pressing down of the sacrum that makes the lifting up of the arms and legs so pleasant.

PRIMARY ADJUSTMENT. One important thing that happens to the lower back in Bow Pose, as in all backbends, is the slight forward movement of the top of the sacrum into the body. This movement is called nutation and passively accompanies extension, or back bending, of the lumbar spine. When nutation is allowed to happen normally, then backbends feel better.

One thing that inhibits nutation is the action of tucking the tailbone. This tucking is the opposite of nutation and makes back bending more difficult. It is impossible to tuck the tailbone in Bow Pose: notice how your student's tailbone lifts off the floor as he or she raises the legs in the pose.

Another way to make sure that nutation can occur is to encourage each student to allow the legs to open to the distance that feels natural. Requiring all students to keep their legs together in the pose will interfere with nutation and can cause lower back discomfort.

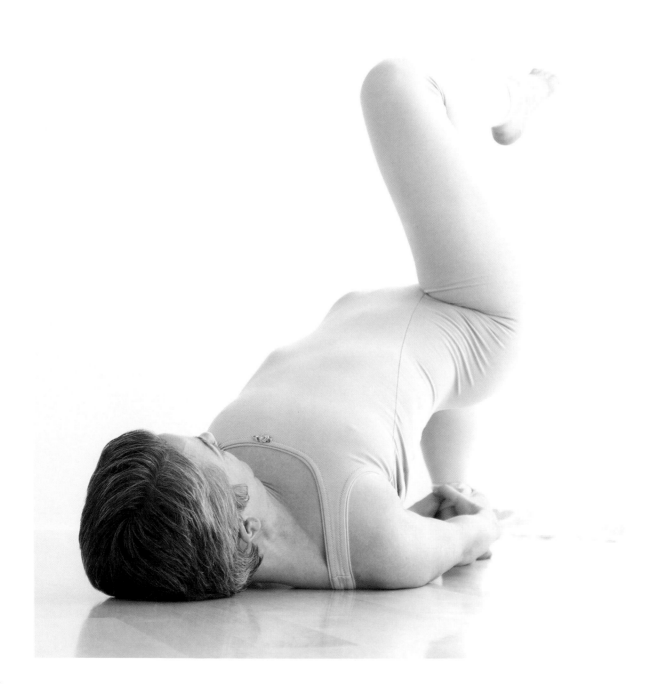

Bridge Pose
Setu Bandhasana

17

A BRIDGE is a connection between two things, such as the two banks of a river. We also speak of *building a bridge:* between people, between cultures, or between countries. In yoga, Bridge Pose (Setu Bandhasana) symbolizes the connection between the inner and the outer world, the mind and the body, and the individual and the Divine. Practice it with joy and release.

SEQUENCING. Bridge Pose can be practiced as part of a backbend series or after Supported Shoulderstand Pose (Figure 20.1)

BENEFITS. Bridge Pose strengthens the erector muscles in the midback and lower back, as well as the muscles between the shoulder blades. It strengthens the legs, especially the hamstrings, the quadriceps, and the buttocks. In addition, this pose stretches the abdomen and the chest muscles; increases the flexibility of the upper back, the shoulders, and the wrists; and counters the effects of sitting for long periods of time.

CAUTIONS. Do not practice Bridge Pose or its variations during menstruation, during the second and third trimesters of pregnancy, or if you have a hiatal hernia. If you have repetitive strain injury (RSI) in one or both wrists, then do not practice Bridge Pose with Yours Hands on Your Back, Fingers In (Figure 17.2).

The Essential Pose *(Figure 17.1)*

PROP: 1 nonskid mat

Spread your mat on a firm and level surface, and lie on your back. With an exhalation, bend your knees, one by one, and place your feet parallel to each other and on the floor, close to your buttocks. Make sure that your shins are vertical.

Exhale and lift your pelvis off the floor by curling up first from your tailbone. Lengthen your pelvis out and away over your legs to elongate the line of your spine. Imagine that your pelvis is moving in one direction and your chest in the other. As you lift, move your arms under your back and interlock your fingers with your arms straight. Keep breathing and gently roll your shoulders under, first one shoulder and then the other.

EXPLORATION. Press your arms into the floor to help you lift. Your arms will act as an anchor to help you roll your shoulders under more, as well as facilitate the opening of your chest. Keep your breathing natural. You may want to take hold of your ankles for a few breaths. Release your hands, breathe quietly, and come down on an exhalation, slowly rolling from the shoulders to the pelvis.

FIGURE 17.1

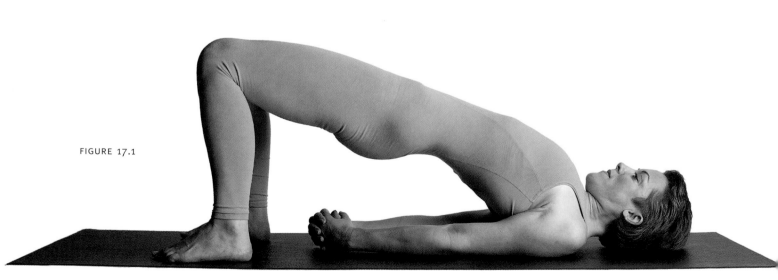

Variations

Props: 1 nonskid mat   ✦   1 bolster

Bridge Pose with Your Hands on Your Back, Fingers In *(Figure 17.2)*. Come into Bridge Pose. As you exhale, bend your elbows, one by one, and roll your shoulders under, placing your hands on your back as close to your shoulder blades as possible. Turn your fingers in and your thumbs toward the sides of your body, so that you can lift your chest even more. Stay in the pose for several breaths, and then release your arms one by one, and roll down with an exhalation.

FIGURE 17.2

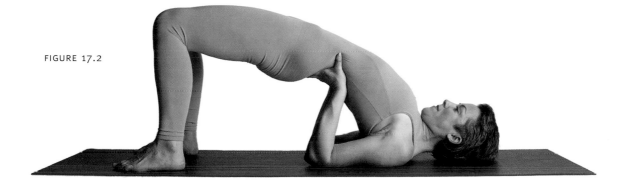

Bridge Pose with Your Hands on Your Back, Fingers Out *(Figure 17.3)*. Come into Bridge Pose. As you exhale, bend your elbows, one by one, and roll your shoulders under. Firmly place your hands around the rim of your back pelvis, with your fingers turned out and your thumbs turned in. Gently use your hands to draw your pelvis away from your chest. Press your elbows down and roll your shoulder blades together to open your chest. Stay in the pose for several breaths. To come out, release your arms and hands, and roll down with an exhalation.

Supported Bridge Pose *(Figure 17.4)*. Few poses are as quieting or relaxing for an agitated mind as Supported Bridge Pose. This variation can reduce blood pressure.

Place your bolster on your mat. Sit on one end and lie back, so that your shoulders are off the edge and lightly touching the floor. Your neck should not be on the floor, but your outer shoulders and upper arms should be. In this position, make sure that your head is on the floor and that your face is parallel to the ceiling. Bend your knees and put your feet on the floor and on either side of the props. Place your arms comfortably out to the sides. Notice the openness of your upper chest. Close your eyes and breathe normally. Stay in the pose for five to ten breaths. To come out, gently roll to the side, lie there for one minute, and then use your arms to help you come to a sitting position.

Especially for Teachers

Prop: 1 strap

Primary Focus. Often when students begin to practice this backbend, they turn the feet out. This happens because of the actions of the glutei maximus. These powerful muscles have two actions: hip extension (which facilitates back bending at the hip joint) and external rotation of the thigh (which causes the feet to turn out).

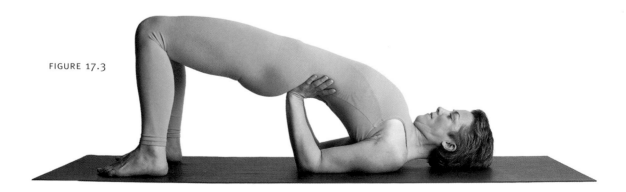

FIGURE 17.3

When a student calls upon the glutei maximus to help in extension, he or she also gets the secondary action of external rotation. The net effect of recruiting the glutei maximus is that the feet turn out. What is happening is that the glutei maximus are working to extend the hip while the adductors are neutralizing the external rotation component of the glutei maximus. It takes training to become aware of this tendency and to learn to keep the feet parallel.

Thus, when you teach your student to keep the feet parallel and the knees over the feet, he or she will be learning to stabilize the pelvis in the backbend. Additionally, he or she will be making it easier for the pelvis to move back over the thighs in a backbend, because the external rotation of the thighs will no longer interfere with that movement. Encourage your student to keep the knees over the feet in this and all backbends.

PRIMARY ADJUSTMENT. When your student understands how to align the feet and knees, try this aid. Using a strap, stand near your student's feet and face her head. After asking for and receiving permission to touch your student, slip the strap around the back of her waist, and pull it snugly around the back rim of her pelvis. Make sure that you, as the helper, are standing upright with your feet in a stable position and your knees slightly bent.

Wrap the loose ends of the belt around your hands so that your elbows are straight. With an exhalation, pull the belt up and back in a diagonal line to help your student lift her pelvis up and away from her chest. Do not lift her off the floor, but give a firm enough lift so that she understands what it means to lift the pelvis toward the knees. Continue to lift the student while you breathe naturally for several breaths. Slowly release the strap and let the student roll down on her own. Repeat once.

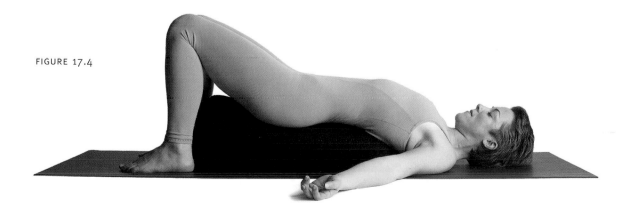

FIGURE 17.4

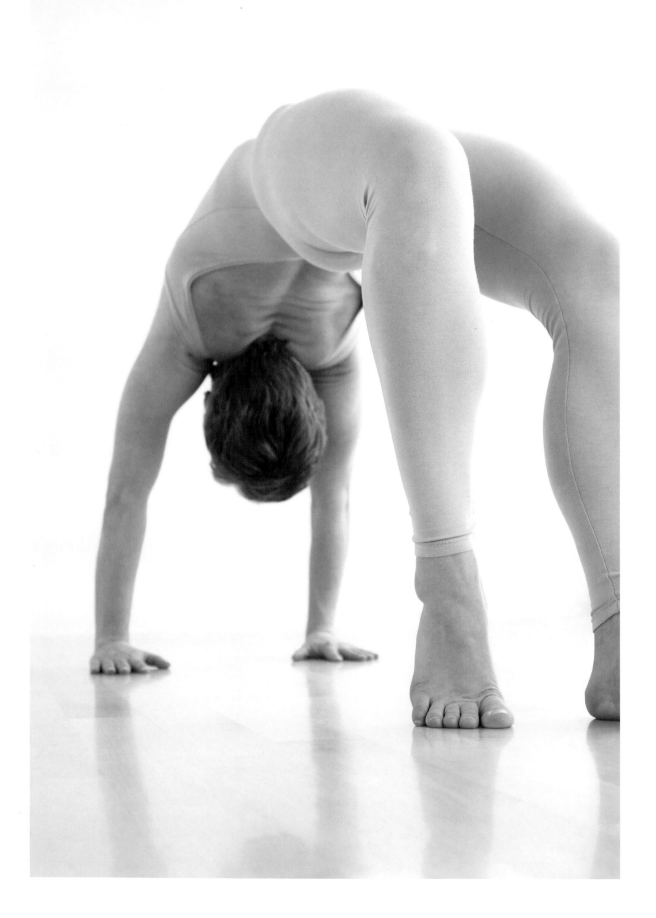

Upward-Facing Bow Pose
Urdhva Dhanurasana

18

WITHOUT A DOUBT, Upward-Facing Bow Pose (Urdhva Dhanurasana) is one of the most beautiful and elegant yoga poses. It requires a perfect balance of flexibility, strength, and courage. It can produce feelings of exhilaration. Practice this pose regularly, with love and persistence.

SEQUENCING. Strong backbends, such as the Upward-Facing Bow Pose, are usually practiced after several standing poses, plus some combination of Lunge Pose (Figure 14.1), Cobra Pose (Figure 15.1), and Bow Pose (Figure 16.1). Do *not* practice it as the first backbend in a backbend series.

BENEFITS. Upward-Facing Bow Pose strengthens the erectors, the hamstrings, and the quadriceps, as well as those muscles in the hips and buttocks, such as the gluteals and the external rotators. This pose stretches the abdomen and chest muscles; increases the flexibility of the upper back, shoulders, and wrists; and counters the effects of sitting for long periods of time. In addition, it can strengthen the bones in the back and help the spine retain its youthful freedom of movement. Research indicates backbends stimulate the bones of the back to retain their calcium, thus helping to prevent osteoporosis in these bones.

CAUTIONS. Avoid this pose and its variations during menstruation, and during the second and third trimesters of pregnancy. If you have repetitive strain injury (RSI) in one or both wrists, then do not practice this pose or its variations.

The Essential Pose *(Figure 18.1)*

PROP: 1 nonskid mat

Spread your mat on a firm and level surface, and lie on your back. Exhale and bend your knees, one by one, placing your feet parallel to each other and on the floor close to your buttocks. Make sure that your shins are vertical.

Place your hands behind you and on the floor. They should be slightly wider than your shoulders; your fingers should point slightly outward. Make sure that your elbows are close to your head and over your shoulder joints. *It is preferable to have your hands wider than your shoulders and your elbows over your hands, rather than your hands close to your head and your elbows falling out.* Press your shoulder blades into your back as you press your elbows inward. Be sure that the bases of your knuckles are on the floor and that your thumbs are opened away from your fingers and pressing down.

Inhale, and with an exhalation, drop the back of your waist to the floor in a pelvic tilt. Then lift your pelvis off the floor by curling up and leading with your tailbone. Do not lift up from your belly, but lead

FIGURE 18.1

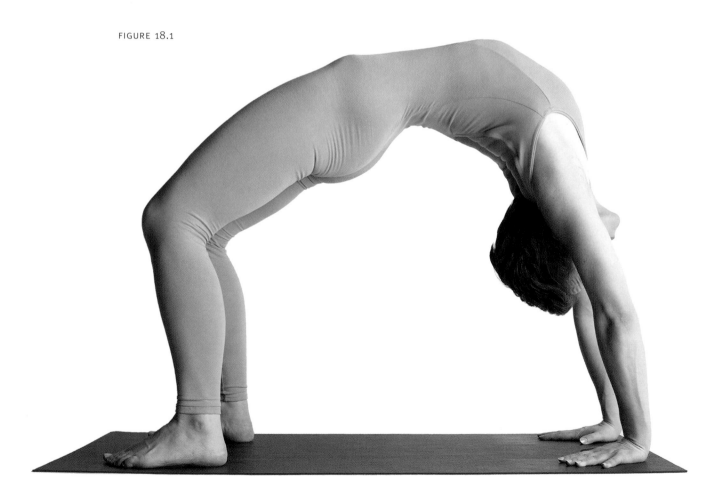

from your tailbone, so that your pelvis is moving out and up in the direction of your knees. To help you do this, push strongly with your hands to move your pelvis in the direction of your feet and to elongate the line of your spine. Keep your breathing fluid and natural.

As your pelvis moves up and your legs straighten, come onto the balls of your feet, making sure that your knees and feet do not roll out. As your knees straighten, your arms will, too. Press your fingers into the floor. As you inhale, lift your breastbone. As you exhale, firmly press your heels down.

Imagine that you are stretching out in all directions from the front of your body as you press down with your hands and feet. Stay in the pose for up to seven breaths. Come down by bending your elbows, place the pelvis on the mat, and then roll down onto the shoulders. Release your arms and take several breaths before repeating the pose two more times.

EXPLORATION. We use the expression "bending over backwards" to describe what it is like to do something difficult. Many adults find Upward-Facing Bow Pose challenging. One of the powerful explorations in practicing this pose is to learn how to make it easier. My recommendation: Stay as relaxed as possible as you lift into the pose.

Because going up into this pose requires a certain amount of strength, a student may often hold the breath, screw up the face, generally tighten up, and then try to push up. When you place your hands and feet in position, take a moment to cool down. Breathe evenly, relax your jaw and tongue, drop your eyes to your lower lids, and let your gaze be receptive. Then begin to tilt your pelvis, and move into the pose with this attitude of *softness*. The *harder* the pose, the more necessary it is to remain *easy and receptive* during practice. When you do, whatever the outcome—whether you do or do not get all the way up—you will enjoy the pose more and benefit from it more if you are relaxed.

VARIATIONS

PROPS: 1 nonskid mat ✦ 2 blocks ✦ 1 wall

UPWARD-FACING BOW POSE AT THE WALL AND WITH YOUR HANDS ELEVATED ON BLOCKS (*Figure 18.2*). Spread your mat on a level, smooth surface, with the long side against a wall. Place the long sides of your blocks securely against the wall. Leave room between them for your head and shoulders. Lie on your back with your head between the blocks. With an exhalation, bend your knees, one by one, and place your feet on the floor. They should be parallel to each other and close to your buttocks, and your shins should be vertical. Position your hands firmly and evenly on the blocks, so that your fingers point toward the center of the room.

Drop the back of your waist to the floor in a pelvic tilt. Then lift your pelvis off the floor by curling up and leading with your tailbone. Do not lift up from your belly, but rather lead from your tailbone so that your pelvis is moving out and up toward your knees. To help you do this, push down with your hands to move your pelvis in the direction of your feet and to elongate your spine. It will take a little more work to get up using the blocks, but they will help your upper back and shoulders open once you can.

As your pelvis moves up and your legs straighten, come up onto the balls of your feet, making sure that your knees and feet do not roll out. As your knees straighten, so will your arms. Inhale and lift your breastbone up and toward the wall. Exhale and firmly drop your heels down. Stay in the pose for three to seven breaths. Come down by bending your elbows, place your pelvis on the mat, and then roll down onto your shoulders.

UPWARD-FACING BOW POSE AT THE WALL AND WITH YOUR FEET ELEVATED ON BLOCKS *(Figure 18.3)*. Spread your mat on a level, smooth surface, with the short side against a wall. Place the short sides of your blocks securely against the wall. Lie on your back, and with an exhalation, bend your knees, one by one, and place your feet on the tops of the blocks.

Come into the pose as previously described. It will take a little more work to get up using the blocks, but using the blocks under the feet will help take pressure off your lower back once you are there. Make sure that your feet press the blocks firmly. As you breathe, lift your breastbone up and out toward the center of the room, and move your pelvis toward the wall. Stay in the pose for three to seven breaths. Come down by bending your elbows, place your pelvis on the mat, and then roll down onto your shoulders

FIGURE 18.2

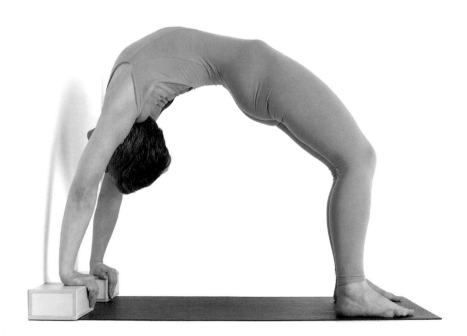

ESPECIALLY FOR TEACHERS

PROPS: 1 to 2 blocks ✦ 1 strap

PRIMARY FOCUS. At first, students roll the feet out as they come into Upward-Facing Bow Pose. This happens, in part, because such a strong action requires the action of all the muscles of the lower body. One set of these muscles is the external rotators of the hip joint.

These muscles, including the piriformis and other muscles, turn the thigh outward during this backbend and other hip extension movements. It takes some practice for the student to learn how to neutralize this external rotation by activating the inner thigh muscles. One way to do this is to place a block the long way or one block the long way and another block the short way between the student's feet before he or she goes up. Then ask the student to press into the block during the process of coming up and holding the pose. This will encourage a strong contraction of the adductors and will keep the rotator muscles from turning the legs and the feet out. Turning the feet out can interfere with the comfort of the lower back in the pose.

Another way to prevent the rotators from acting too strongly in the pose is to offer the student rotator stretches as part of his or her regular practice. For example, the student may try Lying Twist Pose (Figure 27.1) to help stretch this area.

PRIMARY ADJUSTMENT. After your student comes into the pose, sit near his feet. Ask for and receive permission to touch your student. Place a strap around the backs of his knees, and pull horizontally outward. Your pull should be firm yet gentle. As you do this, ask the student to straighten his knees against the pressure of the belt. By doing so, the student will experience his body lifting up and away from the floor. Ask the student to hold this pose for three to five breaths. Then remove the belt so that he can come down with an exhalation.

FIGURE 18.3

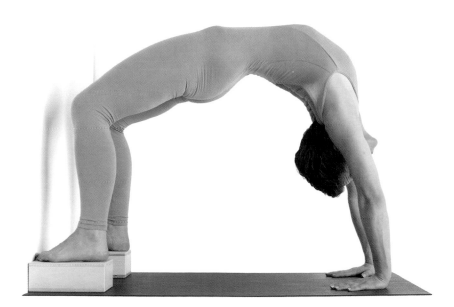

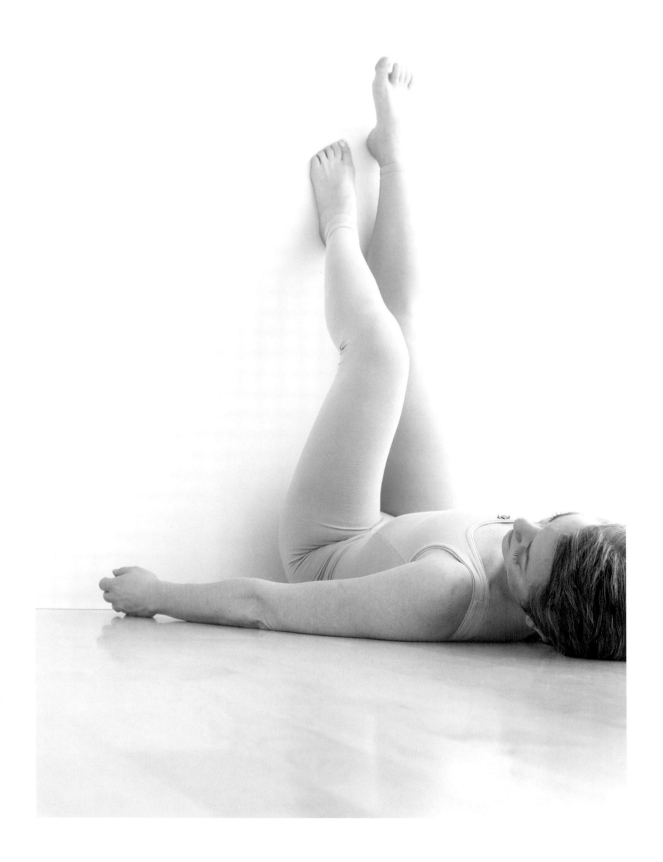

Elevated Legs-Up-the-Wall Pose

Viparita Karani

19

GETTING UPSIDE DOWN every day helps me to see things right side up. Perhaps this is a definition of *perspective*. Practice Elevated Legs-Up-the-Wall Pose (Viparita Karani) not only when you feel tired, but also when you need a fresh point of view. Looking at things from a head-down position can give you a new take on old problems.

SEQUENCING. To center and refresh yourself, practice this inverted pose near the beginning of a quiet yoga session. You can also practice it at the end of your practice before Basic Relaxation Pose (Figure 30.1). Most important, try it by itself during the day when you need to relieve leg fatigue caused by standing or running, or to antidote stressful living, or to experience a brief alternative to a nap.

BENEFITS. Elevated Legs-Up-the-Wall Pose reduces fatigue, lowers blood pressure, and quiets the mind.

CAUTIONS. Do not practice this pose if you are menstruating or pregnant, or if you have glaucoma, a detached retina, a hiatal hernia, or heart problems. Check with your health care professional if you have any concern about elevating your legs.

The Essential Pose *(Figure 19.1)*

PROPS: 1 nonskid mat   ✦   3 blankets   ✦   1 wall

Spread your mat on a firm and level surface, with the short end near the wall. Stack two folded blankets, and place them approximately 8 to 10 inches from the wall. Fold the third blanket in a long shape, and place it on the stack and perpendicular to it.

Coming into this pose may take some practice. If you do not get it right the first time, then give yourself the chance to try it a couple of times. Sit on the edge of the blanket stack with your left shoulder facing the wall. With an exhalation, roll back, swing your legs up the wall, and lie back. Your pelvis should be resting on the blanket stack with your tailbone hanging over the edge near the wall and your last rib just at the front edge of the blankets. The long blanket supports your spine, shoulders, neck, and head.

Close your eyes and breathe normally. To begin, stay in the pose for five minutes. When you are more familiar with it, you may want to increase your time to fifteen minutes. Elevated Legs-Up-the-Wall Pose is not intended to stretch the backs of your legs. If you feel pulling there, then move farther away from

FIGURE 19.1

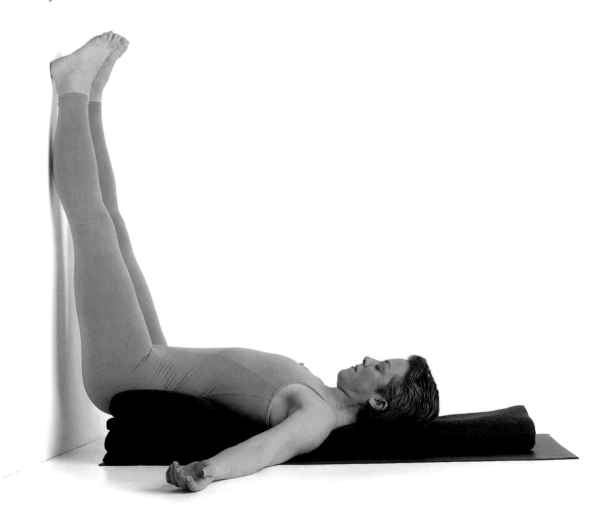

the wall. To come out of the pose, bend your knees halfway toward your chest and roll to the side. Use your arms to help you sit up. Move slowly.

EXPLORATION. Once you are comfortable in the pose, you can deepen your experience by focusing on your breathing. This pose is especially opening for the lungs under the middle and top rib cage. You should be positioned on the blankets so that your lower ribs fall away from each other. This means that your lungs are in a position of openness.

Begin by observing the position of your lowest front ribs. Next, expand your awareness to include observing the natural rhythm of your breath. When you feel comfortable with that, take slow, gentle, and deep inhalations and exhalations. Make sure that the breaths are the same length and that you do not experience any sense of strain or breathlessness. Take twenty of these long breaths, and then let your breathing return to normal. Be present with the sense of calm and equanimity that you feel. When you are ready, bend your knees, roll to the side, and slowly sit up. Remember to use your arms to help you.

VARIATIONS

PROPS: 1 nonskid mat   ✦   3 blankets   ✦   1 wall

ELEVATED LEGS-UP-THE-WALL POSE WITH LEGS IN BOUND-ANGLE POSE *(Figure 19.2)*. Come into Elevated Legs-Up-the-Wall Pose. When you are comfortable, bend your knees out to the sides, and bring the soles of your feet together. Stay in the pose for ten more breaths. To come out, bring your knees together, roll to one side, and use your arms to help you sit up.

FIGURE 19.2

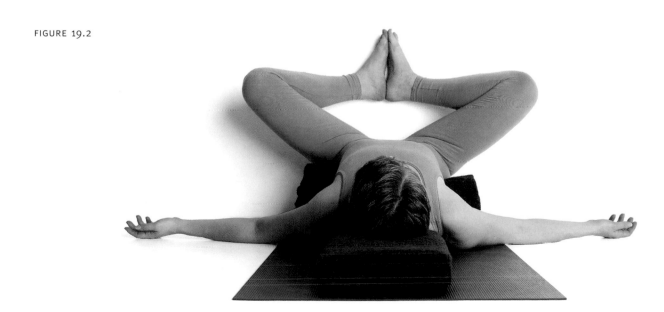

ELEVATED LEGS-UP-THE-WALL POSE WITH LEGS IN SEATED-ANGLE POSE *(Figure 19.3)*. Come into Elevated Legs-Up-the-Wall Pose. Once you are comfortable, open your legs out to the sides. Keep your tailbone dropping down and over the edge of the blankets. Let your knees roll out a little, so that your legs are comfortable. Be sure to monitor your inner knees: if you feel discomfort, then bring your legs slightly closer together. Stay in this pose for eight to ten breaths. Come out by bringing your legs together, bending your knees, and rolling to the side. Use your arms to help you to sit up.

ESPECIALLY FOR TEACHERS

PROPS: 2 pillows

PRIMARY FOCUS. The primary focus in Elevated Legs-Up-the-Wall Pose is comfort. There are three things that you can do. First, students frequently place their props too close to the wall for comfort. Make sure that your student is sufficiently far from the wall to allow the tailbone to drop slightly. A way to be sure of this is to observe your student's abdomen, which should be parallel to the floor, *not* positioned so that the tailbone tilts up toward the ceiling. This position will facilitate comfort in the pose.

Second, suggest alternative arm positions. The arms can be placed to the sides or over the head, with the wrists crisscrossed over each other and resting on the blanket. Be sure to remind your student to reverse this crisscross halfway through the pose.

FIGURE 19.3

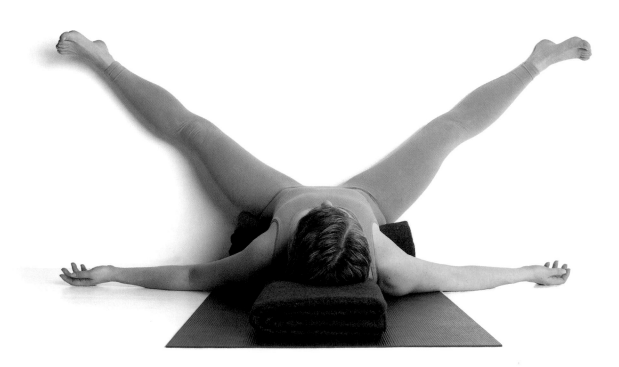

Finally, a student with tight shoulders can use two small pillows, one under each forearm. Position your student's arms out to the sides with the elbows bent at ninety degrees. Then place support under each forearm from elbow to wrist. This may be helpful to a student suffering from neck pain as well.

PRIMARY ADJUSTMENT. It is not uncommon for a student to rest the head with the chin higher than the forehead. There are two reasons to avoid this. First, this position puts too much arch in the neck, which may cause discomfort. Second, this position is often experienced as stimulating to the mind. One of the things that the pose is designed to do is to quiet the mind. Dropping the chin slightly lower than the forehead will help to accomplish this.

To adjust a student, sit or lean over, knees bent, near the top of his or her head. After asking for and receiving permission to touch him or her, slip your hands under the back of the student's head. Inhale and, as you exhale, gently move the student's head toward you, as you gently roll it to drop the chin. Then carefully place the student's head back on the blanket. Slowly remove your hands.

A word about breathing: I find it helpful to remember my breathing as I touch a student. When I stay in contact with my breathing, it helps me to stay present with the student.

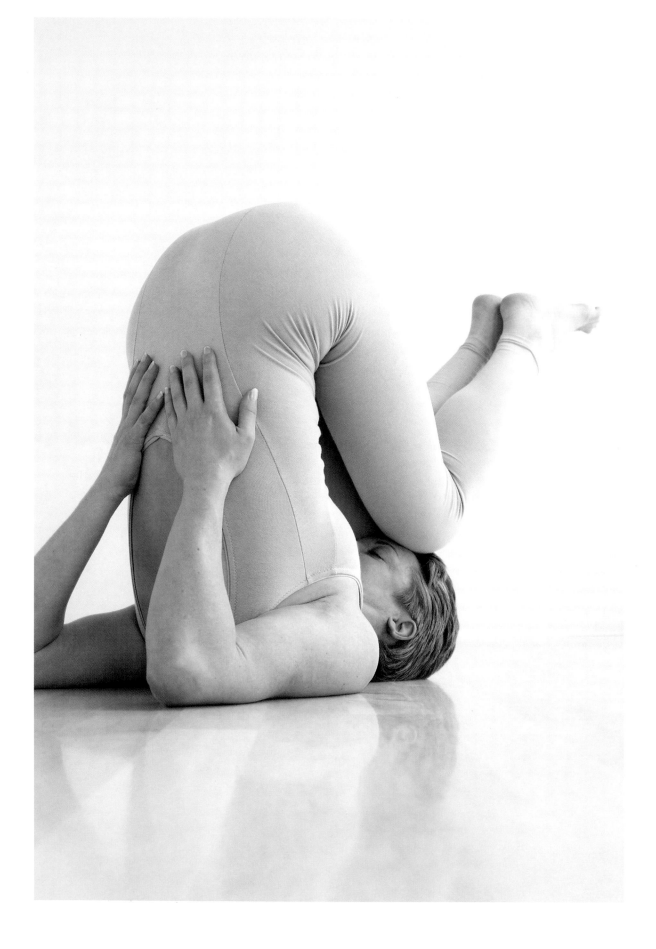

Supported Shoulderstand Pose

Salamba Sarvangasana

20

THE LITERAL TRANSLATION of *Salamba Sarvangasana* is "good-for-all-of-you pose." In addition to what I describe under "Benefits," Supported Shoulderstand Pose offers you a different perspective on your life: when you turn upside down, everything around you looks different. But the world has not changed: you have changed your relationship with it. When you look at the old with new eyes, you put it in perspective, which is the foundation of freedom.

Most people find Supported Shoulderstand Pose challenging in the beginning. Part of putting your life in perspective is in understanding that change happens with time, and it may be in big jumps or in small increments. Remember, it is the process of the pose that is the point, not some idealized goal or performance.

SEQUENCING. Prepare for Supported Shoulderstand Pose by practicing standing poses and simple backbends. Follow it with Downward-Facing Dog Pose (Figure 10.1) or seated forward bends.

BENEFITS. Supported Shoulderstand Pose improves balance, and it drains fluid from the legs and lungs. It stretches the back of the neck and opens the chest. In addition, it can help to lower blood pressure and provide a generalized calming and relaxing effect on your whole body.

CAUTIONS. Do not practice this pose if you are menstruating or pregnant, or if you have neck problems, retinal problems, glaucoma, a hiatal hernia, or heart problems. If you have hypertension, then practice this pose and its variations only under the guidance of an experienced teacher.

The Essential Pose *(Figure 20.1)*

PROPS: 2 nonskid mats   ✦   1 wall   ✦   5 or more blankets

I *strongly* recommend the use of the wall when practicing Supported Shoulderstand Pose. If you are new to the pose, then using the wall will give you confidence and safety as you learn. It is helpful even if you are familiar with the pose, because it helps you to control your ascent and descent.

Place the short side of one mat against the wall. Then fold your blankets and stack them on the mat, positioned approximately 12 to 16 inches from the wall. This distance is individual and it may take some experimentation to find the best distance for you. Put the second mat on top of the blanket stack.

Sit on your blankets with your left shoulder facing the wall. Gently roll back and swing your legs up so that they touch the wall. Your head now rests on the floor, with your chin slightly lower than your forehead. The tops of your shoulders should be about 3 or more inches from the edge of the blankets. This position allows your shoulders to roll toward the edge of the blankets without sliding off as you invert.

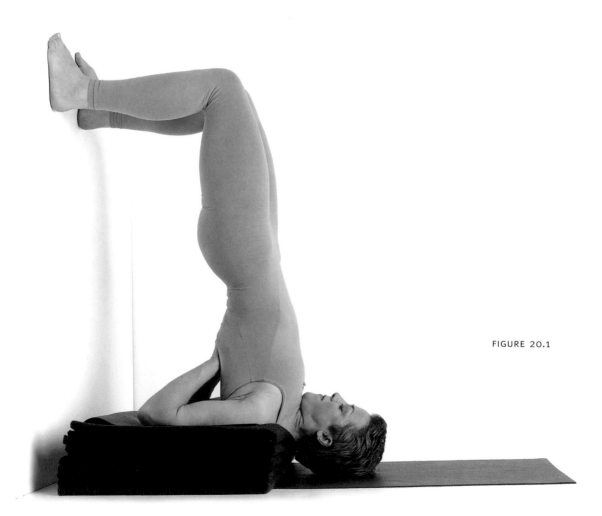

FIGURE 20.1

Inhale and, with an exhalation, press your feet against the wall evenly and lift your pelvis. If the force of your pressure is outward, then you will push yourself off the blankets toward the center of the room. Instead, press your feet against the wall as you simultaneously lift your pelvis, using the strength of your abdominal muscles to *curl up* to vertical. As you lift, clasp your hands behind your back and interlock your fingers. Straighten your arms, stretch them away from your torso, and rest them on the blankets. Keep your breath easy.

Once you are as high up as is comfortable for you, shift your weight to one shoulder, and then gently roll the *other* shoulder under and toward the midline of your body. Repeat to the other side. You should now be resting on the very tops of your shoulders. Bend your elbows and place your hands on your back, with your fingertips pointing toward each other and parallel to your ribs. Try to keep your elbows no wider than the shoulders and pressing down firmly.

The first time that you attempt this pose, stay for five to ten breaths. Gradually work up to five to ten minutes, with your feet lightly but securely on the wall. It might take several weeks or months to stay this long. *There is no rush.* Practice with faith, patience, and ease. Keep your breath easy and your eyes looking softly toward your heart.

Remember, the key to gaining the benefits of this pose is to keep your chest open. This will create the maximum amount of room for your abdominal and thoracic organs, as well as ease your breathing. Throughout the course of days or weeks, *gently* work your hands down your back to lift and open your chest as much as possible. *For stability, be sure to keep both feet on the wall as you move your hands down your back.* Imagine that you are climbing down a ladder instead of up. After moving one hand, exhale and try the other. Pause and take stock of the effects of the new hand position.

To come out of the pose, inhale, and with an exhalation, slowly roll down from your shoulders, first to your waist, and finally to your lower back, so that your upper torso rests on the blankets. Next, wiggle off the blankets so that your shoulders are on the floor, while your lower back and pelvis remain on the blankets. Your head and shoulders should now be completely supported by the floor. Remain here for three to five breaths. Bend your knees, one by one, toward your chest, and gently roll to one side. Inhaling, use your arms to help you sit up.

EXPLORATION. Adjust your blanket height to what feels best to you. You may find that you do better with fewer blankets or that you feel good only by adding more. Do not hesitate to experiment with the number of blankets, even if you have been practicing this pose for years.

But how do you know what you need? Take stock after practicing the pose a couple of times. For example, if you feel your chest dropping or you can't breathe freely, you may do better with four, or five, or six, or even seven blankets.

VARIATIONS

PROPS: 1 nonskid mat ✦ 1 wall ✦ 5 or more blankets ✦ 1 pole

SUPPORTED SHOULDERSTAND POSE WITH A POLE *(Figure 20.2).* If you have tight shoulders, then you may experience two things in Supported Shoulderstand Pose. First, when you place your hands on your back, your elbows may move out to the sides and lift off the blankets. Second, the more you move your hands down your back, the farther the elbows may pop out. These elbow positions leave your back without the necessary support. To solve this problem, you can use a pole. Many students find that this helps them to keep their elbows firmly on the blankets and shoulder-width apart for the first time.

If this is your first experience with this variation, then have someone hand you the pole. With practice, you will be able to place the pole on your blankets before you go up, and learn to pick it up while you are in the pose.

Come into Supported Shoulderstand Pose, and then either pick up or have someone hand you the pole. Hold it with your palms facing toward you, and then press it against your back. The position of your hands does not matter in this variation. You can hold the pole with your hands wide apart, even wider than your back. This will facilitate getting your elbows down and closer together. Beginners can hold for ten breaths. Over time, you can increase the time to five minutes.

To come out of the pose, *keep your feet on the wall for support,* and roll down with an exhalation. Set the pole on the floor in the space between the wall and the blankets.

ONE-LEGGED SHOULDERSTAND POSE *(Figure 20.3).* Once Supported Shoulderstand Pose has become a habit, try the variation called One-Legged Shoulderstand Pose. To begin, come into Supported Shoulderstand Pose. Keeping your attention on your left leg, exhale as you lower your right leg so that it is parallel to the floor, or a little lower if possible, without dropping your chest. Keep your right knee straight: do not allow it to bend in order to take your foot down lower. Remember, the focus is to keep your spine

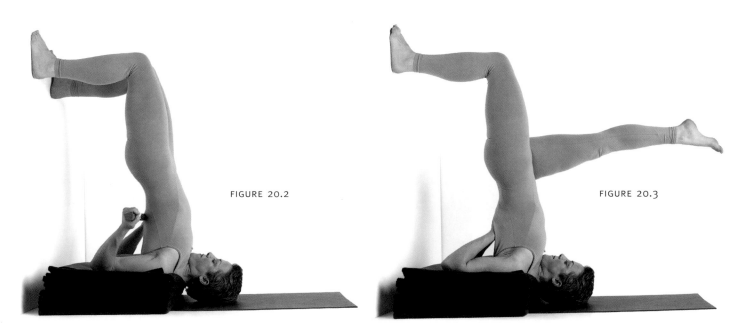

FIGURE 20.2   FIGURE 20.3

undisturbed and your chest open. Take care not to drop the right hip as you lower the leg, but keep it lifted.

Hold the pose for three to five breaths. Then, without disturbing any other part of your body, exhale as you lift your leg back up. Spend a moment re-establishing the position of your spine and your legs. Take a few breaths and then repeat this variation to the other side. To come out of the pose, roll down as previously described.

BALANCING IN SUPPORTED SHOULDERSTAND POSE *(Figure 20.4)*. When you feel stable and secure, which may take several weeks, months, or even longer, practice Balancing in Supported Shoulderstand Pose by taking one foot and then the other away from the wall to balance freely. When you do this, place your feet together, straighten your legs, and lift upward through them toward the ceiling. Hold for as many as ten breaths, gradually increasing your time in the pose to five minutes. To come out of the pose, lower your legs, one by one, and place them on the wall. Roll down as previously described.

ESPECIALLY FOR TEACHERS

PRIMARY FOCUS. It is critical to teach Supported Shoulderstand Pose and its variations in a way that protects the student's cervical spine. The normal cervical spine flexes only about 75 degrees, not 90 degrees as some may assume. The blanket support will help the student keep the neck flexed at a healthful angle, as well as prevent the weight of the body from coming down directly onto the cervical bones and overstretching the posterior cervical ligaments. Using the blankets for support is a safer way to practice and one that honors the student's anatomy.

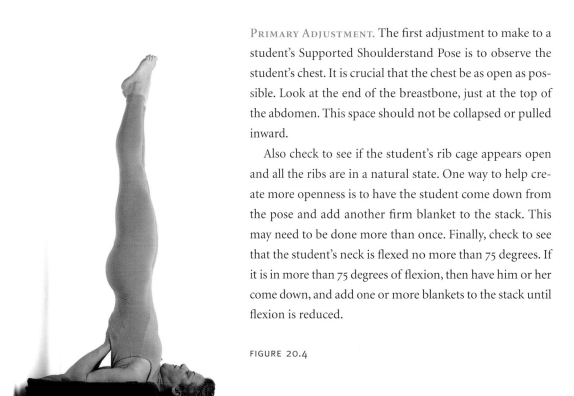

PRIMARY ADJUSTMENT. The first adjustment to make to a student's Supported Shoulderstand Pose is to observe the student's chest. It is crucial that the chest be as open as possible. Look at the end of the breastbone, just at the top of the abdomen. This space should not be collapsed or pulled inward.

Also check to see if the student's rib cage appears open and all the ribs are in a natural state. One way to help create more openness is to have the student come down from the pose and add another firm blanket to the stack. This may need to be done more than once. Finally, check to see that the student's neck is flexed no more than 75 degrees. If it is in more than 75 degrees of flexion, then have him or her come down, and add one or more blankets to the stack until flexion is reduced.

FIGURE 20.4

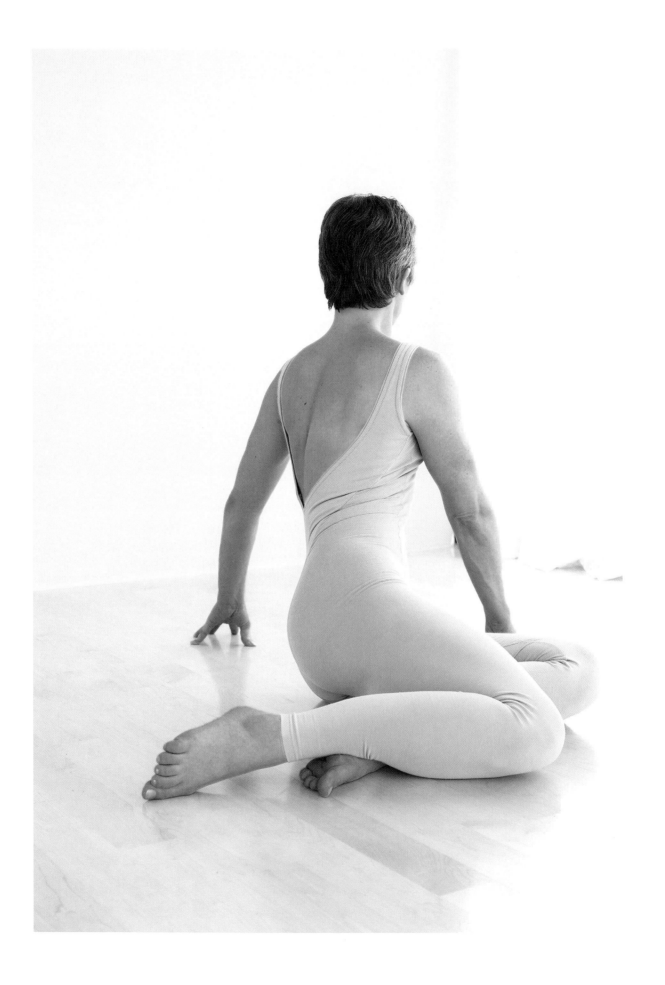

Simple Seated-Twist Pose
Bharadvajasana

21

SOMETIMES LIFE TWISTS YOU into knots. Simple Seated-Twist Pose (Bharadvajasana) is a gentle way to *un*twist the spine and the mind. This pose can help to refresh your back muscles after long bouts of sitting, and will provide a bit of stimulation when you are feeling sleepy or dull.

SEQUENCING. You can practice this twist after a series of backbends and before attempting other poses. It can also be used after a series of forward bends to relieve any residual lower back discomfort. Do not use Simple Seated-Twist Pose as your last pose before Basic Relaxation Pose (Figure 30.1). The movement is too asymmetrical for the spine to be practiced before lying down to relax.

BENEFITS. Simple Seated-Twist Pose increases the flexibility of the spine, improves breathing by stretching the intercostals and opening the chest, and stimulates the abdominal organs.

CAUTIONS. Do not practice this pose if you have diagnosed disc disease in your lower back. If you are pregnant, then do not strongly contract your abdominal muscles as you twist: instead twist gently, allowing your belly to remain soft.

The Essential Pose *(Figure 21.1)*

PROPS :   1 nonskid mat   ✦   1 blanket

Place your mat on a smooth, level surface. If needed, you can sit on a folded blanket for comfort. Have your legs in front of you. Bend your knees and swing your legs to the left so that you are sitting, for the most part, on your right hip. Place your left lower leg and ankle area into the arch of your right foot. Separate your knees about 10 inches to 1 foot. This distance really depends on your comfort. If you are comfortable with your legs closer together, then practice the pose that way.

If you feel that you are leaning to the right, if you are uncomfortable, or if your left hip is off the ground, place a firmly folded blanket under your *right* hip and buttock to lift the right side of your pelvis to the same height as the left (see Figure 21.1a).

Before you twist, make sure that your pelvis is as level as possible. Remember, the pelvis is the base of the spine, and the stability and evenness of your pelvis will help to create an enjoyable pose.

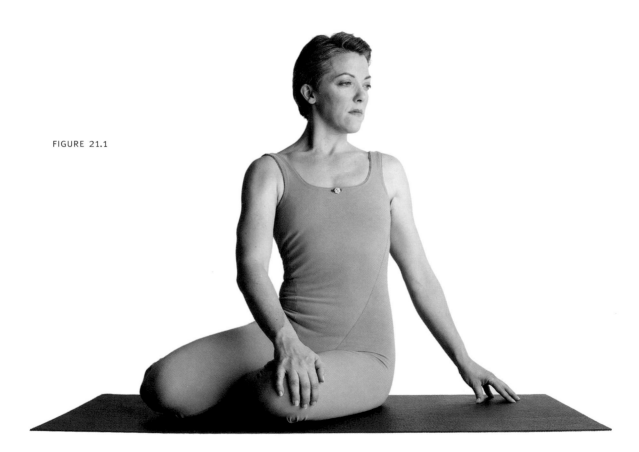

FIGURE 21.1

Reach across your body with your left hand, and hold the outside of your right knee. Place your right fingertips on the floor behind you for support. Inhale, and with an exhalation, draw your abdominal muscles strongly into your belly, and then twist around to the right from the base of your pelvis to the top of your head. In this new position, inhale, and with the next exhalation, draw the belly in again and twist even more. Keep your shoulders level. Although your left pelvis may lift slightly, it is important to keep your left thigh firmly anchored to the floor. Think of your pelvis as part of your spine and thus let it move; think of your left thigh as the foundation of the pose.

As soon as you feel resistance to the twisting movement, stop, breathe, and let your body adjust to the new position. Often you will be able to twist gently to the right some more. Take several exhalations to twist gradually around. When you have twisted around as much as you enjoy, stay there for several breaths before coming out of the twist. Then repeating the twist. When you have finished twisting to the right twice, practice the twist to the left two times.

FIGURE 21.1A

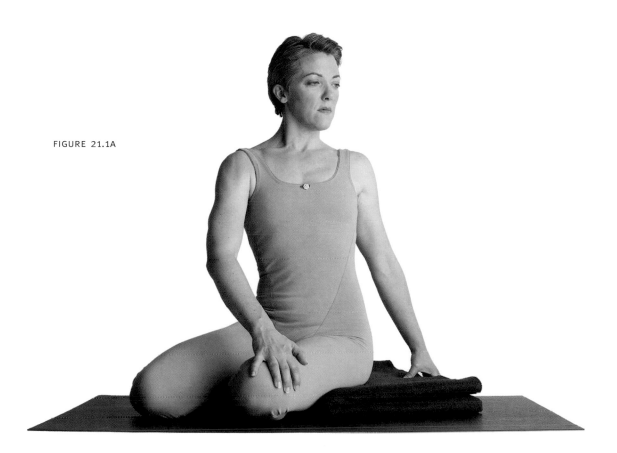

EXPLORATION. Experiment with head placement. You can either turn your head into the direction of the twist, or you can turn it in the opposite direction. You may find it difficult to twist your body in one direction while twisting your head in the other. At first, this will take concentration and awareness, which are two hallmarks of yoga practice.

Whichever position you choose, turn your head and allow your gaze to follow. Sometime students aggressively turn their eyes into the twist instead of building the pose from the base and letting the upper body, neck, head, and eyes receive the twist.

VARIATION

PROPS: 1 nonskid mat   ✦   1 blanket   ✦   1 wall

SIMPLE SEATED-TWIST POSE AT THE WALL *(Figure 21.2)*. Place the short side of your mat near the wall. Sit on a folded blanket, with your right shoulder about 10 inches away from and parallel to the wall. Come into Simple Seated-Twist Pose with your legs to the left, and twist to the right. Inhale, and with the

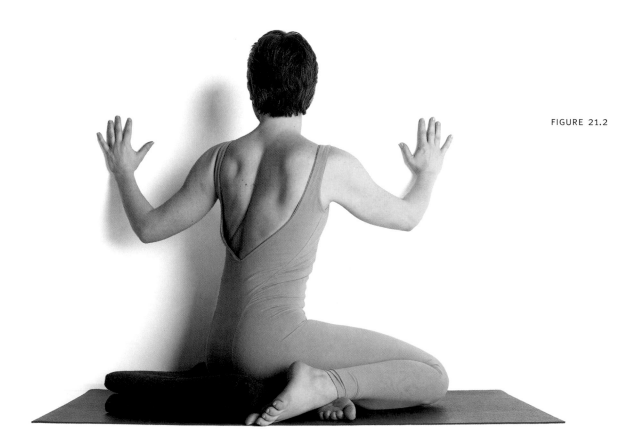

FIGURE 21.2

exhalation, lift your right arm out in front of you, and bend your elbow as you stretch over your head in a circle. Place your right hand on the wall slightly behind you and at eye level. Place your left hand on the wall at eye level as well. Both elbows are bent at a right angle. Inhale, and with an exhalation, press with your right fingertips to push yourself into the twist, all the while pressing with your left fingertips to push yourself away from the wall. Do not lean into the wall as you twist. Repeat it a second time to the right before practicing it two times to the left.

ESPECIALLY FOR TEACHERS

PRIMARY FOCUS. Many students have difficulty understanding the separation that can be felt at the hip joint of the back leg in this twist. Most students tend either to keep the pelvis and thigh on the floor or to lift both. Keeping both the thigh and the pelvis down forces the spine to move independently from the pelvis and can create some strain in the sacroiliac joint. This is the place where the spinal column and the pelvis are connected. It is subject to strain in twisting motions if the pelvis and the spine do not move together.

Lifting both the thigh and the pelvis also has consequences. It does not allow the student to have a sense of grounding from which to lift. Encourage your student to press down on his or her thigh while allowing the pelvis to lift into the twist. This is the best of both worlds: your student experiences the stability created by the thigh, as well as the freedom and safety of the pelvis moving with the spine to deepen the twist.

PRIMARY ADJUSTMENT. This adjustment will help your student to understand separating the movement at the back hip joint. Ask for and receive permission to touch her. Then stand slightly behind your student, and place your hand on her upper thigh. If she is twisting to the right, then press on the upper left thigh, right next to where it joins the body. Place your fingers toward you and your inner wrist in the direction of your student's head. With an outward rotational movement, press with just enough force to feel her skin spinning toward you and down the outside of her thigh. This is the direction of external rotation.

Combining the pressure to ground her thigh as you simultaneously externally rotate it will help your student understand exactly where to lift from her pelvis to increase the twist. Never push your student deeper into a twist by moving her shoulders. This can be harmful to the back. Rather, help your student understand the twist by providing her with a clear experience of the foundation of the pose so that she can fly upward in a delicious spiraling movement.

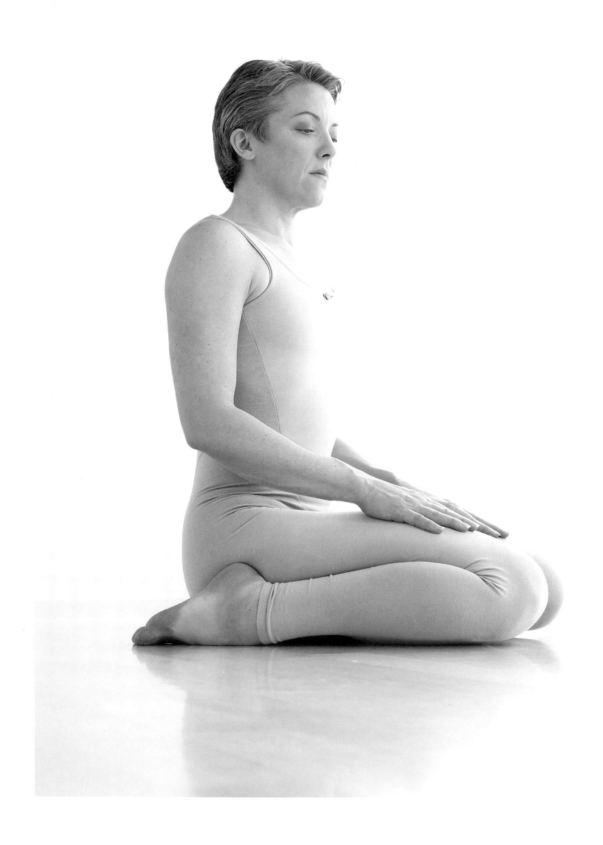

Hero–Heroine Pose
Virasana

22

IN MANY PARTS of the world, Hero–Heroine Pose (Virasana) is a classic sitting posture, one that is sometimes used for meditation. However, many Westerners find this way of sitting on the floor unusual and hard on their knees. Do not let the fact that this pose is unusual deter you from including it in your regular practice. Practice it every day until you are more familiar with it. Proceed with caution and consistency, and you will create or regain youthful flexibility in your knees and thigh muscles.

SEQUENCING. Before you practice Hero–Heroine Pose, first practice several standing poses and Standing Forward Bend Pose (Figure 11.1).

BENEFITS. Said to be beneficial for digestion, Hero–Heroine Pose also helps to create flexibility in the feet, ankles, knees, and quadriceps.

CAUTIONS. Hero–Heroine Pose is a paradox. Although it is not recommended for those who have any variety of knee injuries or undiagnosed knee pain, many students have found that it can help cure these very dysfunctions. Therefore, if you have significant knee pain or a knee injury, then practice this pose *only* under the guidance of an experienced yoga teacher. Do not stay in the pose for more than three to five breaths if you suffer from varicose veins in your legs. Finally, some women in the last trimester of pregnancy find that their knee ligaments are too loose for them to practice comfortably, or that their thighs or lower legs are too swollen for them to enjoy the pose for more than just a couple of breaths.

The Essential Pose *(Figure 22.1)*

PROPS: 1 nonskid mat   ✦   2 blankets

Place your mat on a firm and level surface. Fold one blanket so that it measures 2 feet by 18 inches and kneel on it. Sit back on your heels and take several breaths. *If this preliminary action is difficult in any way, then come out immediately. Instead, practice Hero–Heroine Pose, Sitting on a Block (Figure 22.2).*

If sitting on your heels is comfortable, then lift up enough to allow you to use your hands to pull your outer upper calf muscles away from your thighs, one by one, before you sit down between your heels. Make sure that your knees are one fist-distance apart and that your toes are pointing straight back and not out to the sides.

You may occasionally see children sitting in Hero–Heroine Pose, with the feet turned out so that the arches of the feet are on the floor. This can exert an extreme stretch on the inner knee ligaments. Although

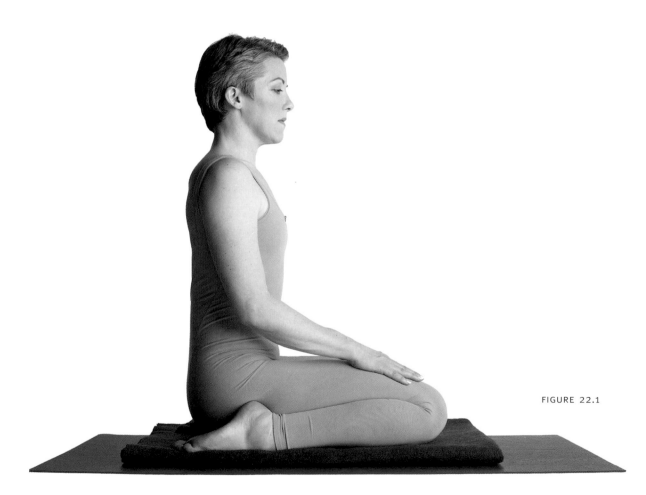

FIGURE 22.1

children may feel comfortable in this position, it can permanently overstretch the inner knee ligaments: it is not recommended. Luckily, adults usually find this movement of turning the feet out in the pose painful or impossible. But make sure that you are turning your feet so that the soles of your feet point upward toward the ceiling, thus helping to maintain the integrity of your knee joints.

Once you are in the pose, carefully reassess your body. You may want to rise up slightly and place the second blanket at the back of your knees and thighs before you sit down again (see Figure 22.1a). You will need to experiment with the thickness of this folded blanket. This adjustment can give some space to the knees and may be enough to alleviate any discomfort. Place your hands on top of your thighs and keep your breath easy. Stay in the pose for five to ten breaths.

To come out of the pose, lean forward onto your hands and bring your weight onto your hands and knees. Gradually straighten your knees, walk back, and stand up with an inhalation. This way of coming out of the pose will minimize any torque in your knees.

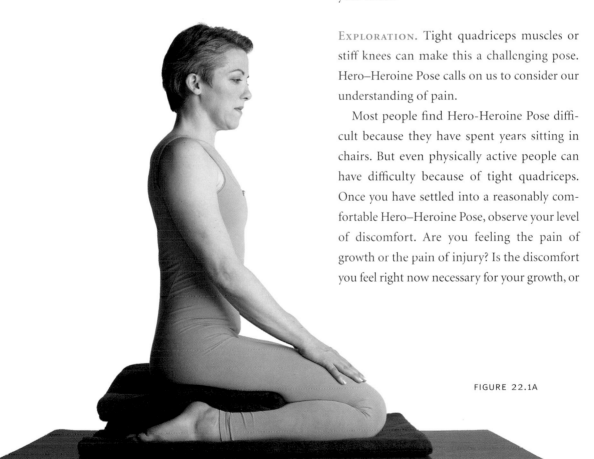

EXPLORATION. Tight quadriceps muscles or stiff knees can make this a challenging pose. Hero–Heroine Pose calls on us to consider our understanding of pain.

Most people find Hero-Heroine Pose difficult because they have spent years sitting in chairs. But even physically active people can have difficulty because of tight quadriceps. Once you have settled into a reasonably comfortable Hero–Heroine Pose, observe your level of discomfort. Are you feeling the pain of growth or the pain of injury? Is the discomfort you feel right now necessary for your growth, or

FIGURE 22.1A

is that sensation of discomfort a signal from your body and mind warning you to listen and to act?

Knowing the difference between these two kinds of discomfort is wisdom. Life presents you with difficulties. But if you run from the difficulties, you will not be able to live. So the question to be answered if your life is to be rich and full, concerns not how to avoid pain, but rather *which* pain to avoid. Establish this discrimination in Hero–Heroine Pose and keep it with you throughout your yoga practice. It is an invaluable understanding to take off your mat and into your daily life.

VARIATIONS

PROPS: 1 nonskid mat ✦ 1 block ✦ 3 or more blankets

HERO-HEROINE POSE, SITTING ON A BLOCK *(Figure 22.2)*. Set up your mat and blanket as for Hero–Heroine Pose. Kneel down and place the block between your heels. Make sure that you adjust your calves and, if you need it for comfort, add a folded blanket behind your knees. Stay in the pose for at least five to ten breaths. If you are a beginning student and find this variation comfortable, then you can gradually increase your time in the pose. Even if you are an experienced student, you will enjoy this variation; you may be able to stay in the pose for long periods or use this variation for meditation. Come out by leaning forward onto your hands and bringing your weight onto your hands and knees. Gradually straighten your knees, walk back, inhale, and stand up.

HERO-HEROINE POSE WITH ARM STRETCH *(Figure 22.3)*. Including this variation in your practice will not only stretch your shoulders, but will give you a way to lengthen your time in the pose. You may enjoy the combination of Hero–Heroine Pose for your lower body and this shoulder stretch for your upper body.

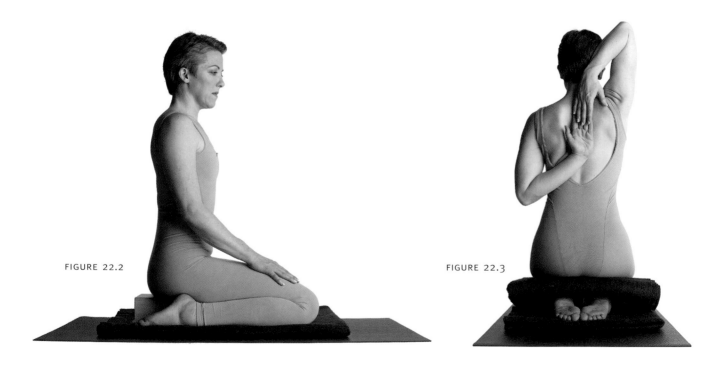

FIGURE 22.2

FIGURE 22.3

Begin by setting up your mat and blanket as for Hero–Heroine Pose. Adjust your calves and, if necessary for comfort, add a folded blanket behind your knees. With an inhalation, stretch your left arm out to the side and about 14 inches away from your body. As you exhale, quickly bring your arm behind you and place your forearm on your spine, so that the back of your hand touches your back.

Wiggle your left arm up your back, toward your collar, as far as you can without strain. Inhale, and lift your right arm overhead. As you exhale, bend your right elbow and clasp the fingers of your left hand or, if possible, your full left hand. Roll both of your shoulders back to keep them open at the front. Make sure that you are not tilting your rib cage, shoulders, or spine to one side. Keep your rib cage and shoulders parallel to the floor and your spine long and centered. Hold this arm stretch for about five breaths before releasing. Try it one more time before practicing it on the other side.

ESPECIALLY FOR TEACHERS

PROPS: 1 low bench   ✦   1 bolster   ✦   1 block   ✦   3 or more blankets

PRIMARY FOCUS. The primary focus of Hero–Heroine Pose is the health and safety of the knees. Encourage your student to practice Hero–Heroine Pose only after fully stretching the knees out straight in a pose such as Standing Forward Bend Pose (Figure 11.1).

Most Westerners are not used to sitting in this position, and so it should be approached with caution. Encourage your student to begin with the variation called Hero–Heroine Pose, Sitting on a Block (Figure 22.2) before taking the full pose. Remind him or her of the foot position: soles pointing up, toes pointing back, and little toes down.

If a student with high arches experiences foot discomfort, then suggest that the student practice on a bed until he or she is more comfortable in the pose. Occasionally, I have suggested that a student sit on a low bench or on a bolster. This allows the student to sit in the pose with very little weight on the knees.

PRIMARY ADJUSTMENT. If your student complains of mild knee discomfort in the pose, then help him to turn the upper calves out and hold this position *while* he sits down. Your student can do this by sitting on the heels, raising up about 6 to 8 inches, grasping the very tops of the calves in the bend of the knee, and turning and holding the outward pull *as* he sits down again.

Additionally, your student can try dragging the flesh of the back upper calves toward the heels at the same time that he turns the upper calves out. These adjustments seem to free most knees for Hero–Heroine Pose. However, I have found that sometimes dragging the calf muscles inward instead of outward has helped to relieve discomfort.

It is important to remember that a little discomfort during the pose is probably fine. However, if discomfort in or around the knees is felt after the pose or even after class, then the student should modify Hero-Heroine Pose by sitting higher on the block, by sitting on a stack of blankets or a bolster, or by sitting on a low bench the next time.

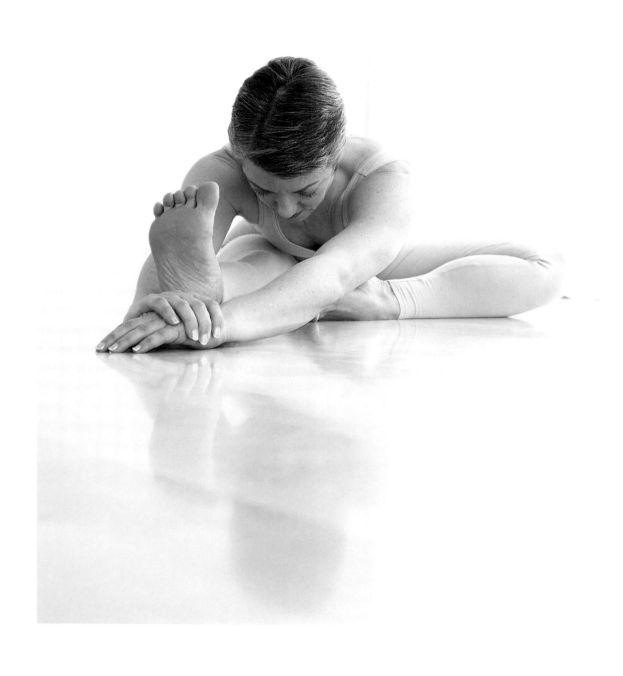

Head-of-the-Knee Pose
Janu Sirsasana

23

IN A YOGA CLASS, Head-of-the-Knee Pose (Janu Sirsasana) is often the first seated forward bend taught to new students. Although this pose will definitely challenge most beginners, more experienced students can find it interesting as well. But remember, what makes this a yoga pose is *not* that you can touch your toes: it is *staying present* on the way down.

SEQUENCING. Head-of-the-Knee Pose usually is practiced near the end of a class, after standing poses and Standing Forward Bend Pose (Figure 11.1). It can also be practiced with good effect after seated twisting poses.

BENEFITS. Head-of-the-Knee Pose stretches the hamstrings in the back of the straight-leg thigh and also the lower back muscles, especially those on the same side as the bent knee. It also increases flexibility in the hip joint on the same side as the bent knee. It can quiet the belly organs, lower blood pressure, and help the mind to turn inward. I especially recommend this pose for menstruating and pregnant women.

CAUTIONS. Do not practice this pose if you have diagnosed disc disease in your lower back. Practice this pose with extreme care if you have knee pain or a significant knee injury, and then *only* under the supervision of a qualified yoga teacher.

The Essential Pose *(Figure 23.1)*

PROPS: 1 nonskid mat   ✦   1 blanket

Place your mat on a firm and level surface, and place a folded blanket on the mat. Sit close to the edge of the folded side of the blanket, with your legs straight out in front of you. Bend your right knee about halfway toward your body, and place your right foot on the floor. Place three fingers of your right hand behind the right knee, and feel the hollow there. Exhale, and bend the knee more as you gently pull the flesh of your upper calf and lower thigh out and toward your other leg. This movement will create more space in the back of your knee joint.

Let your right knee drop out to the side and remove your hand. Keep your breath even. Place your right foot about two-thirds of the way between the knee and the groin of your left leg, so that your right shin is perpendicular to your left leg and your right knee points to the right. Now place the fingertips of your left hand behind you, and use your left arm to help you sit upright. Keep your left leg rotating slightly inward, so that there is more weight on your left inner heel than your left outer heel. Turn your left knee slightly inward as well, so that you are resting on your inner left calf and inner left thigh. Gently pull the flesh of your left buttock out toward the left side to increase the feeling that you are actually resting on

FIGURE 23.1

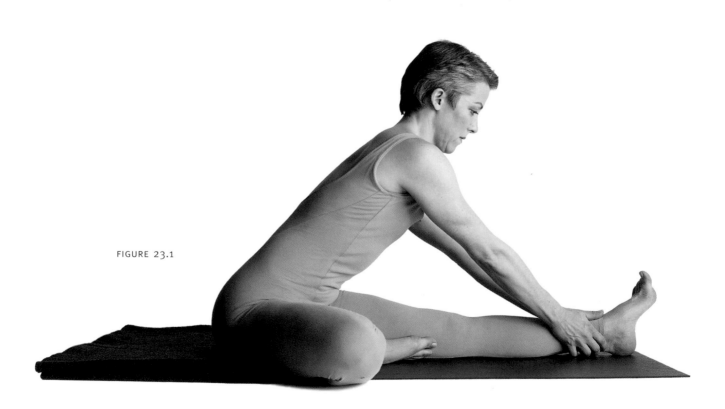

your sitting bones. Remember, the bending movement in all forward bend poses comes from the hip joints moving around the top thighbones, and not from the spine rounding.

Exhale, reach across your body with your right hand, and hold the outside of your left knee, calf, ankle, or foot. Once again, it is very important that this movement be accomplished by tilting your pelvis forward and not by rounding your lower back. Rounding your lower back backward in this flexion movement can put hundreds of pounds of pressure on the discs between your lumbar vertebrae. To prevent this, practice the pose with all bending movements coming from your pelvis moving over your hip joints, thus leaving your spine relatively undisturbed. It is not more spiritual or better to hold the foot rather than the knee. Please practice in this very moment, that is, within your ability, and with an attitude of exploration and curiosity about what is possible for you right now. Just sitting upright with your pelvis tipped slightly forward can be enough, even in flexible people, to create a stretch in the hamstrings.

Drop your head, breathe normally, and gradually stretch out and over your straight leg, rather than thinking of moving down. Avoid the common tendency of bending your left knee in order to get down farther. When you have come to a place of firm but not unbearable stretch, take hold of your foot with both hands. Stay in the pose for five to ten breaths, and come up on an exhalation. Repeat the pose on the right side before switching to the left.

EXPLORATION. Many yoga students decry the resistance they find in their hamstrings when they begin practicing forward bends, especially seated ones. But this resistance is actually the key to practicing yoga. This may seem like a paradox at first glance. Letting go in a forward bend is symbolic of the letting go, of the *viragya,* which the ancient yoga texts, such as the Yoga Sutra of Patanjali, say is necessary to reach the state of wholeness.

The texts teach you to let go of your attachments: your attachment to being right, to having total control, or to living forever. This process of letting go is integral to the process of becoming whole. Most important, the resistance that you feel to letting go, whether it be to letting go of your rigid beliefs or of your hamstrings, is the starting point for your learning.

It is the resistance that creates the possibility of letting go. When you practice this pose now, instead of thinking of the tightness, or resistance, in your hamstrings as the problem, reframe that resistance in your mind as the teacher. Your hamstrings are telling you exactly where you are holding on and exactly where to let go. Emotional resistance serves the same function. In fact, each asana provides you with another opportunity to let go of what is holding you back. Practice Head-of-the-Knee Pose with this awareness, and you will find that the tightness in your hamstrings actually shapes your practice instead of hinders it.

Variations

Props: 1 nonskid mat   ✦   1 to 2 blankets   ✦   1 towel

Head-of-the-Knee Pose with a Rolled Blanket Under Your Bent Knee *(Figure 23.2)*. Set up as for the essential pose. If your bent knee does not reach the floor easily or if you are recovering from a knee injury, then place a rolled blanket under the root of that thigh to offer firm support to the knee. If a rolled blanket is too thick, use a rolled towel instead. When the prop is in place, continue your practice of the pose. Be sure to do two things. First, use the prop when practicing on the other side, even if that side does not require it. This will keep the stretch even for both hip joints. Second, practice the pose for an equal amount of time on both sides.

Head-of-the-Knee Pose with Your Foot Back *(Figure 23.3)*. Because the leg position in this variation makes the pose more challenging, practice it *only* if you can bend forward with ease. Set up as for Head-of-the-Knee Pose. Keep your breath even. Now move your right foot about 6 to 8 inches away from your inner groin, so that your knee is pointing in a diagonal angle toward the back of the room. Remember the anchor of the pose, and as you come forward, firmly but gently press your right shin and thigh into the floor. Practice twice on the right side before switching to the left side.

Especially for Teachers

Props: 1 or more blankets

Primary Focus. Inevitably, the beginning student will want to touch her toes in this pose. Somehow, we all feel more holy if we do, regardless of how we may distort the body to create the stretch.

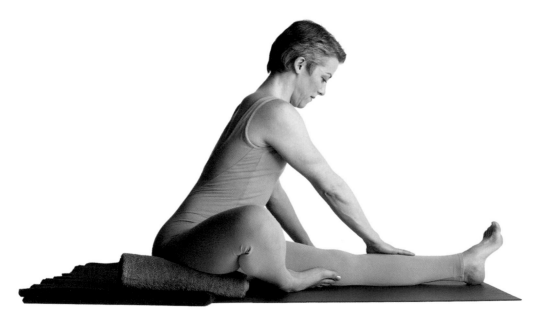

FIGURE 23.2

It is important for the health of your student's lower back that you pay particular attention to the harmony of her lower back and her pelvis. From the very start, teach her to move the pelvis first and let the spine follow. Some beginning students will feel the stretch just by learning to sit upright with the pelvis tilted forward a minimal amount. This position is infinitely preferable to having your student bend forward with the spine rounding and collapsing, almost moving backward in the pose. Be liberal in encouraging your student to sit on as high a stack of folded blankets as necessary to allow the pelvis to tilt forward properly, thus preventing injury.

As your student comes into the pose, her lumbar curve should remain as concave as possible. Remember, a concave arch is actually the neutral position for the lumbar spine. Teaching your student to move in this way will help to prevent lower back pain and dysfunction, especially in the sacroiliac region.

PRIMARY ADJUSTMENT. To further the basic understanding of the pelvis moving independently over the thighbones, try this adjustment. After your student has assumed the first part of the pose, but before she has gone down, kneel behind her bent leg. After asking for and receiving permission to touch her, place one or both of your hands on the back of her upper thigh, near where it meets the torso. Make sure that your thumb points toward the front of her body and that the rest of your fingers point back and down toward the floor. Your thumb should come no farther forward than what is now the highest part of her thigh. *Under no circumstances should your hand touch her inner thigh.*

Inhale, and with an exhalation, press firmly back and down to roll her thigh back and down, thus facilitating external rotation of the hip joint. Your pressure will help her feel that the thigh is in contact with the floor. This, in turn, will help her to differentiate this downward movement from the forward and upward movement of the pelvis. Understanding the movement of the thigh and the movement of the pelvis is the key to enjoying forward bends.

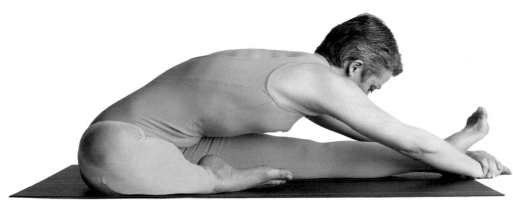

FIGURE 23.3

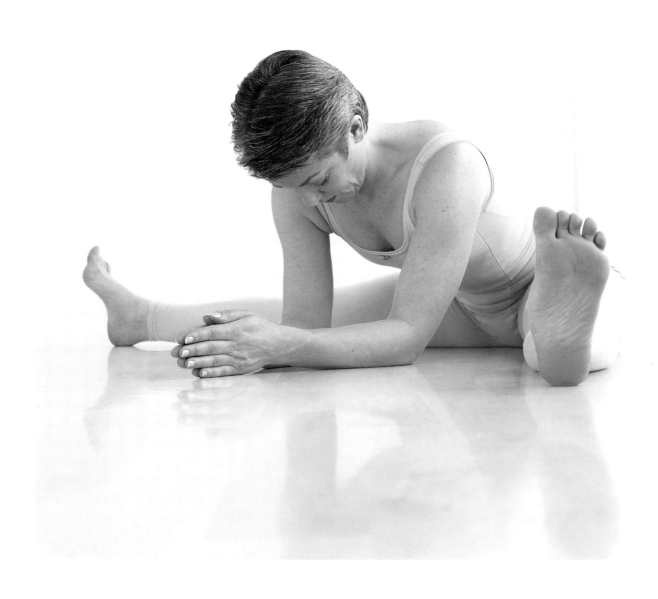

Seated-Angle Pose
Upavistha Konasana

24

IF YOU SPEND A LOT OF TIME sitting in chairs with your legs close together or crossed, then it is likely that you have tight adductors. As a result, you may find Seated-Angle Pose (Upavistha Konasana) difficult at first. This pose requires a level of flexibility in the hip joints and thigh muscles, such as the adductors, that can be challenging. Practice it several times a week, not only to challenge yourself, but also to increase your flexibility. This newfound flexibility will help you to enjoy many of your other poses.

SEQUENCING. As part of a seated series, Seated-Angle Pose usually follows Head-of-the-Knee Pose (Figure 23.1) and can be practiced before or after Bound-Angle Pose (Figure 25.1).

BENEFITS. This pose stretches the adductors and the hamstrings, and increases mobility in the hip joints. It is beneficial for women, especially during pregnancy and menstruation. Supported Seated-Angle Pose (Figure 24.3) can help alleviate menstrual cramps and quiet the mind.

CAUTIONS. Avoid this pose if you have any strain in your inner thigh muscles. Do not bend forward in this pose if you have diagnosed disc disease in your lower back.

The Essential Pose *(Figure 24.1)*

PROPS: 1 nonskid mat ✦ 1 or more blankets

Place your mat on a firm and level surface, and sit down. Separate your legs as wide apart as you can without causing discomfort in your inner knees. Keep your knees straight throughout the pose.

Remember, in all forward bend poses, the bending motion does *not* come from rounding the spine. It comes from tilting your pelvis forward and moving it over the thighbones, thus leaving your spine relatively undisturbed. Rounding your lower back is a flexion movement that can put hundreds of pounds of pressure on the discs between the lumbar vertebrae. Please practice within your ability and with an attitude of exploration and curiosity about what is possible for you right now.

If you can easily lift your spine and maintain its normal curves, then bend forward slowly, breathing with ease and using your arms and hands to support you. Make sure that your knees are straight and that your kneecaps are pointing up. Keep your spine long as you initiate the forward movement from your hip joints and pelvis, and let your spine follow. Gradually stretch forward and keep your breathing easy and relaxed. Enjoy your pose.

If you find that, as you sit on the floor, your pelvis rolls backward, then use props to help you. Fold one or more blankets into a rectangle that measures approximately 2 feet by 18 inches, and stack them. Sit on the firm side and separate your legs. If your spine still is rolling backward or is collapsing at the waist, then put your hands behind you on the floor, press down with your fingertips, and lift your spine gently against that downward movement. Concentrate on rolling your pubic bone slightly forward toward the floor and on lifting your spine and chest. Remember to keep your knees firm and your kneecaps pointing toward the ceiling throughout.

FIGURE 24.1

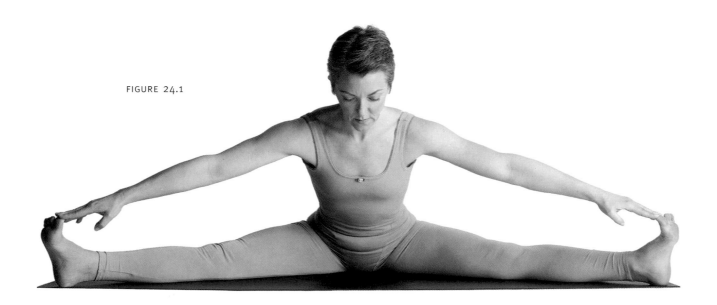

Whether you choose to bend forward or remain upright, stay in the pose for five to ten breaths, come up slowly, and then repeat. To come out of the pose, sit up, lean back slightly, and catch the back of each knee with the corresponding hand. Slowly bend each knee toward you, and place the soles of your feet together in front of you in preparation for the next pose, Bound-Angle Pose (Figure 25.1).

EXPLORATION. There are a couple of ways to explore Seated-Angle Pose. The first way is appropriate for all levels of practitioners. To begin, set up for the pose, sit on your mat (and blankets if you are using them), and separate your legs. As you exhale, turn your torso to the right, so that your breastbone is in line with your right leg. Place your right hand behind you and your left hand between your legs. Inhale, and with an exhalation, draw your belly in and press your fingertips against the floor to help you lift and twist your spine even more toward the right. Let your belly lead the movement. Keep your breath soft. Feel the opposing movements: your left leg stretches out, presses down, and stays stable, in contradistinction to your spine and belly twisting and moving.

As you release your belly and twist to the right, allow your pelvis to come with you, even letting your left pelvis lift slightly off the floor without disturbing your left thigh. Remaining present in the midst of these two opposing forces is a form of training for your daily life. Can you remain stable and yet yielding in the midst of the many contradictions that you find just in living life with your family, your friends, and your coworkers? Hold this pose for five breaths, and then derotate and practice it to the other side.

The other way to deepen your exploration of this pose is more appropriate if you can bend forward easily from your pelvis. If you can do this, then focus on slowly coming forward until you feel the slightest sensation of stretch in your legs. This might be only a couple of inches, so pay very close attention to what you feel in your legs. As soon as you feel any sensation, stop and wait for your body to let go of that resistance. As soon as you no longer feel that resistance, then begin to move very slowly forward again, repeating this slow movement forward, stopping, breathing, and waiting for the body to adapt before asking it to bend any more.

Not only will this way of going into the pose slow you down, but it will remind you of how often you demand that your body do what you want without paying attention to what you are feeling at the time. It will also remind you that resistance in life often can be overcome by your willingness just to be present with that resistance. You don't need to do anything but be present and breathe, and the body will change. Perhaps this skill of waiting and being present with resistance can occasionally be of help in your daily life.

Variations

Props: 1 nonskid mat   ✦   1 or more blankets   ✦   1 bolster   ✦   1 chair

Seated Angle Pose with a Chair *(Figure 24.2)*. This variation is calming and may help to soothe a headache. Position one or more folded blankets on the mat, which you have stacked and placed in front of the chair. (Make sure that the chair cannot slide. However, do not place the chair on the mat, because it could tear the mat.) Separate your legs as wide apart as you can without causing discomfort in your inner knees. Keep your knees straight throughout the pose. If your pelvis is rolling back, then sit on one or more folded blankets.

Fold your arms and put them on the seat of the chair. Rest your forehead on your arms. Close your eyes and breathe slowly. Make sure that the back of your neck rounds slightly and does not sag into an arch. Stay in the pose for ten breaths, and with an inhalation, come up slowly. Sit up, lean back slightly, and catch the back of each knee with the corresponding hand. Then slowly bend each knee toward you, and place the soles of your feet together in preparation for the next pose, Bound-Angle Pose (Figure 25.1).

Supported Seated-Angle Pose *(Figure 24.3)*. Practice this variation if you are comfortable in Seated-Angle Pose and do not need the blankets to help you rotate your pelvis.

Set up as for Seated-Angle Pose. Place the bolster between your legs, close to your body. With an exhalation, bend forward and rest on the bolster. Slip your hands, palms up, under the bolster so that the end supporting your head is slightly elevated. Turn your head to one side, rest on your cheek, close your eyes, and breathe softly. After five to ten breaths, turn your head so that you are resting on your other cheek.

To come out of the pose, use your arms to lift your torso as you inhale. Sit straight up, lean back slightly, and catch the back of each knee with the corresponding hand. Then slowly bend each knee in toward you, and place the soles of your feet together in front of you in preparation for the next pose, Bound-Angle Pose (Figure 25.1).

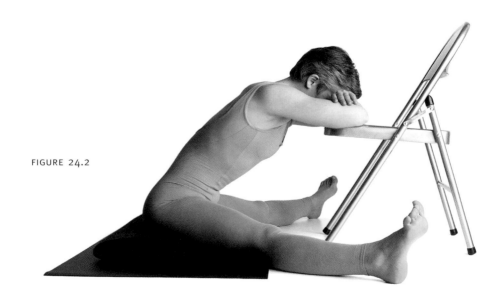

FIGURE 24.2

ESPECIALLY FOR TEACHERS

PRIMARY FOCUS. The virtues of alignment and patience are what is primary in teaching this pose to beginning students. Often they think that the goal is to get the legs as wide apart as possible. Make sure that they do not place the legs so wide apart that it would be impossible for them to reach their toes even if they had the adequate leg flexibility to do so. If necessary, encourage beginning students to *do less*.

It is also common for many students to allow their knees to roll outward or backward. This action stretches the hamstrings unevenly. Remind your student to keep his or her kneecaps pointing to the ceiling.

Finally, it is critical that your student understand the need to bend forward from the pelvis and not from the lower back. This is often difficult to teach in Seated-Angle Pose because so many people have done this stretch before, and are sure that they know how to do it. An infatuation of bending forward at any cost to the lumbar spine can create strain on the intervertebral discs and other soft tissue surrounding the spine. Make sure that your student practices with an adequate blanket height, so that he or she moves from the hip joints. Learning this action is where the practice of patience comes in.

PRIMARY ADJUSTMENT. Ask your student to sit in Seated-Angle Pose. Stand behind him with your right hip and right shoulder facing his back. After asking for and receiving permission to touch the student, place your right outer lower leg against his sacrum and along his spine. Hold each upstretched wrist in each of your hands. As you both exhale, roll onto the ball of your right foot, and press your lower leg in and up against his sacrum. The combination of the pressure of lifting the sacrum and lifting the arms will give him a delicious sensation of lightness and openness in the pelvis. Watch as the lower back lifts and curves gently inward. Hold this adjustment for several breaths, and let go slowly.

Throughout the adjustment, make sure that you as the teacher are in a comfortable position, standing in a stable manner on your left foot and leg and with your spine upright. Remember that when you touch your students, you communicate your attitude powerfully. In fact, he may remember your attitude more than whatever movement the touch was intended to facilitate.

FIGURE 24.3

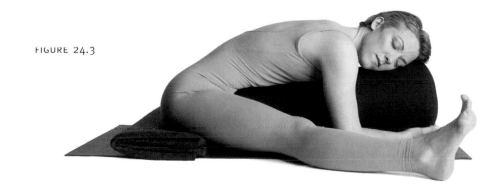

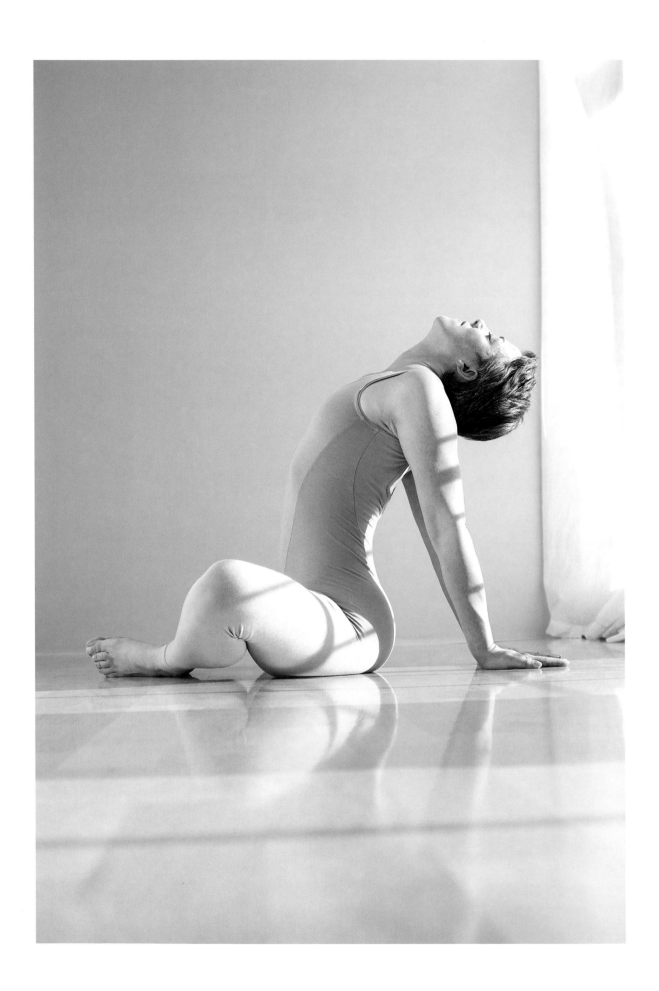

Bound-Angle Pose
Baddha Konasana

25

BOUND-ANGLE POSE (Baddha Konasana) is one of the basic sitting positions of yoga. It is also called Cobbler's Pose, because it is the position that shoemakers use in India. They hold the shoe with the feet, so that both hands are free to work on the shoe that they are making. Westerners can find this pose challenging because of the years we spend sitting in chairs with our knees close together.

SEQUENCING. Practice Bound-Angle Pose before or after Seated-Angle Pose (Figure 24.1) or just before Basic Meditation Pose (Figure 29.1).

BENEFITS. Bound-Angle Pose stretches the adductors and relaxes the abdomen. It may be experienced as soothing to digestive and eliminative organs. It is also believed to have a healthy effect on the uterus of the menstruating and the pregnant woman. I recommend that a pregnant woman practice it every day to facilitate an easier delivery.

CAUTIONS. Be careful of your inner knees when you practice this pose. Do not practice this pose if you have chronic strain or pain in your inner knees or in your inner thigh muscles.

The Essential Pose *(Figure 25.1)*

PROPS: 1 nonskid mat ✦ 1 or more blankets

Place your mat on a firm and level surface, and sit down with your legs out in front of you. Bend your right knee about halfway toward your torso. Firmly place three fingers of your right hand and, as you exhale, bend your knee completely, gently pulling the flesh of your upper calf and lower thigh out toward your other leg. This will create more space in the back of your knee joint.

Let your right knee drop out to the side and remove your hand. Keep your breath even. Place your foot near your pubic bone at the center of your body without pulling it in tightly. Now repeat this process with your left knee, placing the sole of your left foot against the sole of your right foot. Let your knees fall to the side easily.

Notice if your spine is dropping and your lower back is rounding. If this is happening, then insert the corner of a folded blanket under your hips to elevate your pelvis but not your legs. This will relieve your back and simultaneously help your knees drop down toward the floor. If you find that your spine is still dropping and that you are folding at the front waist, then add another blanket. Remember, you want the front of your body to open.

FIGURE 25.1

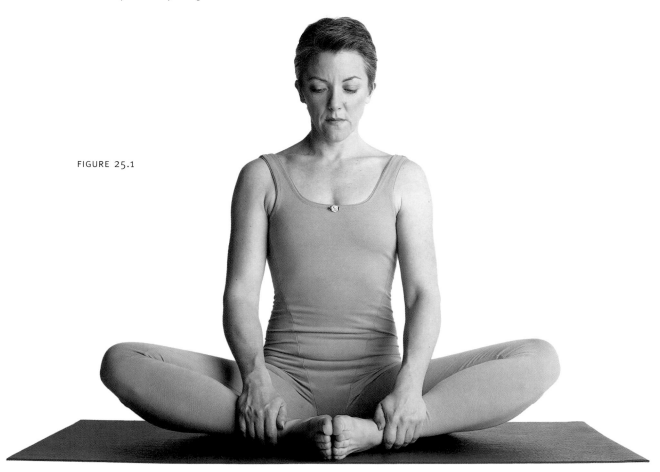

You can do several things with your hands. You may choose to interlock your fingers and hold your feet. If you do so, then do not pull your toes up. Or if your knees are not on the floor and your pelvis tends to roll back in the pose, then put your fingertips on the floor behind you, press firmly, and lift your spine up. Remember to breathe softly. Do not bounce your knees up and down, but instead let gravity pull them down gradually. If your knees are down on the floor and you are easy in the pose, then you may want to bend forward. Do this only if your pelvis and not your spine is initiating the movement.

You can stay in Bound-Angle Pose for long periods of time, but begin by staying no more than one to two minutes; try it while watching TV or folding the laundry. To come out of Bound-Angle Pose, use your hands to help you lift your knees up, and then stretch your legs straight out in front of you as you exhale.

EXPLORATION. To practice yoga is to become aware of your habits, both physical and mental. Use your practice time to explore new ways of moving, feeling, and being in the world. Do not repeat the poses in the same order and the same way every time.

To change your experience of this pose, practice it with your feet at varying distances from your body. Come into the pose as detailed previously, but this time place your feet about 6 inches farther out than the original instructions suggest. Stay in that position for several breaths. If your knees are down on the floor and you are easy in the pose, then you may want to bend forward. Do this if your pelvis and not your spine is initiating the movement. Keep your breath easy and remember to exhale when you bend forward.

Now come up and, this time, place your feet in a different relationship to your body than before. Again, remember to breathe and come forward only if that is appropriate for you. Pay attention to the different sensations of stretch that arise when you change your leg position. Practicing with this spirit of exploration will help you keep your practice alive and interesting.

VARIATIONS

PROPS: 1 nonskid mat ✦ 2 or more blankets ✦ 2 towels ✦ 1 block

BOUND ANGLE POSE WITH ROLLED BLANKETS UNDER YOUR KNEES *(Figure 25.2)*. Set up as for Bound-Angle Pose. If your knees do not reach the floor, then you can place a rolled blanket (or towel) under each knee. When you do, make sure that you do not roll back with your pelvis, but maintain your pelvis and spine in an upright position. Gradually reduce the height of the blankets. Stay in the pose for five to ten breaths, and then come out of the pose with an exhalation.

BOUND ANGLE WITH A BLOCK BETWEEN YOUR FEET *(Figure 25.3)*. Set up as for Bound-Angle Pose. Place the block between your feet. This will change the relationship between your thighs and pelvis, and will create a different stretch in your inner thighs and hip rotators at the outer thigh. Stay in the pose for five to ten breaths, and come out with an exhalation.

ESPECIALLY FOR TEACHERS

PRIMARY FOCUS. The key to this pose is pelvic position. When the student's pelvis rolls backward, the sockets of his or her hip joints roll forward and up. This tends to lift the thighs up and away from the floor. It is critical that your student understand the importance of rolling the pubic bone down toward the floor. This will turn the hip sockets forward and down, and make it easier for the thighs to drop.

FIGURE 25.2

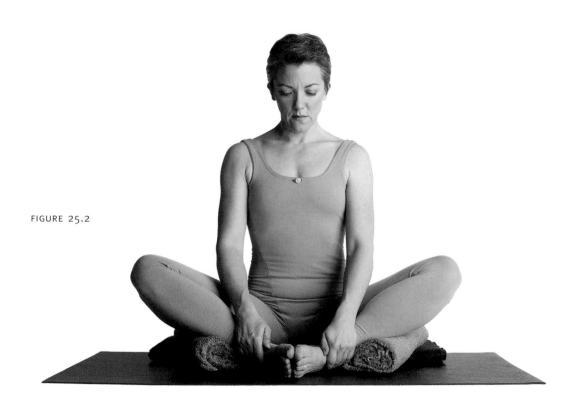

If sitting up on the edge of a couple of folded blankets does not help drop the knees, then the difficulty may be coming from tightness in the hip flexor muscles. Suggest that your student practice Lunge Pose (Figure 14.1) and its variations to stretch this area. The student can try the Lunge Pose immediately before practicing Bound-Angle Pose.

PRIMARY ADJUSTMENT. After your student has assumed the first part of the pose, but before she has bent forward, kneel behind her. After asking for and receiving permission to touch the student, place your hands on the back of her upper thigh, near where the thigh joins the torso. Make sure that your thumb points toward the front of her body and that the rest of your fingers point back and down toward the floor. Your thumb should come no farther forward than what is now the highest part of her thigh. *Under no circumstances should your hand touch the student's inner thigh.*

Inhale, and with an exhalation, press firmly back and down to roll her thigh back and down, thus facilitating external rotation of the hip joint. Your pressure will help the student feel like her thigh is more connected with the floor. This, in turn, will help the student differentiate this downward movement of the thigh from the forward and upward movement of the pelvis. Understanding the independent movement of the thigh and the pelvis is the key to enjoying forward bends.

FIGURE 25.3

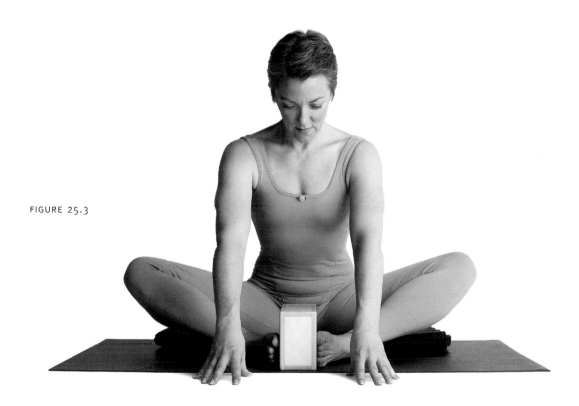

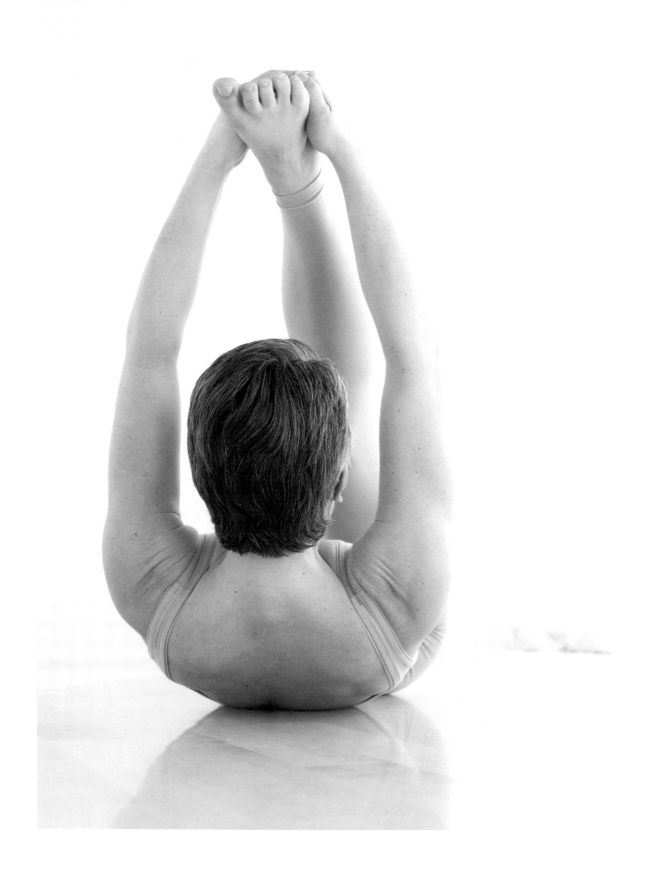

Reclining Leg-Stretch Pose

Supta Padangusthasana

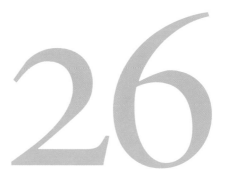

RECLINING LEG-STRETCH POSE (Supta Padangusthasana) is both an effective stretch and a relaxing movement. Whether you sit for many hours a day or are an athlete, you can benefit from the increased hip mobility and hamstring stretch that it provides.

SEQUENCING. Practice this pose first if you are not feeling enthusiastic about starting your yoga session. It will get you going and ease you into a longer practice.

Reclining Leg-Stretch Pose is also an enjoyable pose to place at the end of a yoga session, especially when it is practiced following forward bends. Reclining Leg-Stretch Pose can be practiced after back-bends if you practice a seated twist in between. If you are particularly tired, then include this pose as the beginning of a very quiet practice.

BENEFITS. This pose stretches the hamstrings and the lower back muscles, and helps to create flexibility in the hip joints.

CAUTIONS. Do not practice this pose if you have a hamstring injury or diagnosed sciatica. Also do not practice this pose while lying on your back after the midpoint of pregnancy. In this case, prop up your torso at a 45 degree angle.

The Essential Pose *(Figure 26.1)*

PROPS: 1 nonskid mat   ✦   1 blanket

Spread your mat on a firm and level surface, and lie down. You can place a folded blanket under your head and neck, but this is not mandatory. Do so only if your neck is uncomfortable, or if your chin lifts and your head hangs back.

Align your body so that it is in a straight line. Place your legs together, with your kneecaps facing the ceiling. Inhale, and with an exhalation, raise your right leg. Keep both knees straight and your left leg on the floor. Roll your left leg inward slightly, so that your inner heel presses against the floor.

Once your right leg is up, reach out with both hands, and hold either the back of your knee, your calf, your ankle, or your foot. Be careful not to bend either knee in the attempt. Choose instead the alignment of keeping your knee straight rather than the superficial gratification of bending your knee in order to catch your ankle or foot. Make sure that your shoulders rest evenly on the floor. If either knee bends, then practice Reclining Leg-Stretch Pose with a Strap (Figure 26.2) instead.

FIGURE 26.1

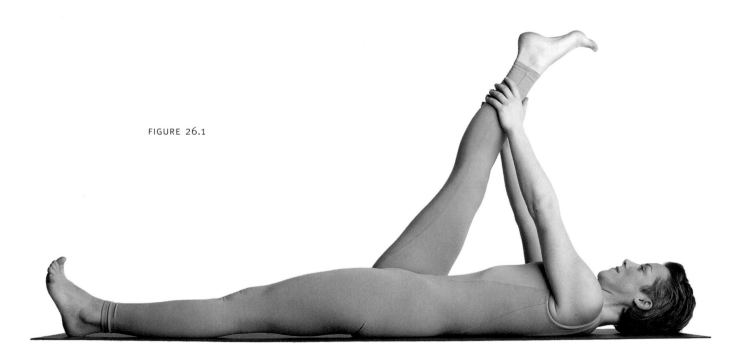

A word about the hamstrings: At one end, three of the four heads of the hamstring attach to the sitting bone, which is located in the bottom of the pelvis. The other head attaches directly to the back of the thighbone. At the other end, they attach to the back inside or the back outside of the knee joint. This makes the hamstring a two-joint muscle. Therefore, in order to stretch it effectively, the muscle must be stretched over both the back of the sitting bone as well as over the knee joint. If you bend your knee to hold the foot or ankle, then you will lose the stretch of the hamstrings. Keeping your knee straight may cause your leg not to come up as high, but it is a more effective way to stretch. Remember, it is not the range of motion that makes the movement a yoga pose: it is, rather, the insight and awareness that you bring to the movement.

Once you are holding onto your leg, inhale again, and with each exhalation, bring the leg farther toward your face. Do not force the leg past the point of a healthy, strong, but still pleasant stretch.

After three to five breaths, lower your leg to the floor with an inhalation. Once your leg is back down, realign your body before practicing Reclining Leg-Stretch Pose to the other side.

EXPLORATION. When you are comfortable in the pose, place your right thumb where your right thigh meets your torso. Your thumb should face in, and your fingers should wrap around the outside of your thigh. With an exhalation, firmly press in as you rotate your upper thigh outward. As you rotate the thigh, press your thumb outward, in a direction that is parallel to the floor, that is, so that you are pressing down and out toward your left foot.

Continue to breathe easily and to use your left hand to draw the leg toward your face. Hold this pose for several breaths before releasing your grip on the back of your knee, calf, ankle, or foot, and lower your right leg with an exhalation. Pressing the thigh down and rotating it out helps to change the relationship of your thigh with your hip socket, and thus changes the experience of the stretch in the backs of the legs. Be sure to practice this exploration on the other side.

VARIATION

PROPS: 1 nonskid mat   ✦   1 blanket   ✦   1 strap

RECLINING LEG-STRETCH POSE WITH A STRAP *(Figure 26.2)*. Come into Reclining Leg-Stretch Pose. Bend your right knee and place a strap over the arch of your foot. Hold an end of the strap in each hand. Use the strap to pull your leg toward your face. Do not bend your knee in the attempt. When your elbows start to bend, move your grip higher on the belt. Make sure that your shoulders remain relaxed. Keep your chin dropped down.

ESPECIALLY FOR TEACHERS

PRIMARY FOCUS. In this pose, it is common for the student to put more focus on the lifted leg. Remind him or her to put equal, if not more, focus on the leg that is on the floor. The student should press down and out through the inner heel of that leg. This point is related to the wider practice of poses. It is easy for the mind to be drawn to movement, but concentration is enhanced when you focus on what is *still*.

FIGURE 26.2

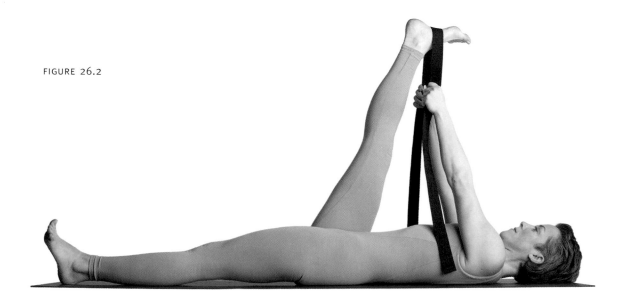

PRIMARY ADJUSTMENT. Have your student practice the pose. Ask for and receive permission to touch him or her before you proceed further. Stand on the outside of the leg that is to be lifted. With both of your hands, firmly hold the student's leg, just below the knee. Exhale while you lift his or her leg about 4 inches off the and externally rotate it. Gently set the leg down in the new position, that is, with the knee rolled out slightly. This will cause the knee to turn out as well as lengthen the side of the waist. The student can proceed with the pose with that leg and hip joint positioned in this new direction. Follow with the adjustment on the other side.

Be sure to ask your student to exhale as you make this adjustment. You will find it helpful to exhale at the same time. This will help you, as the teacher, to stay present with the student and the adjustment, as well as with your own body. In this way, you will learn to avoid injuring yourself as you teach and make adjustments.

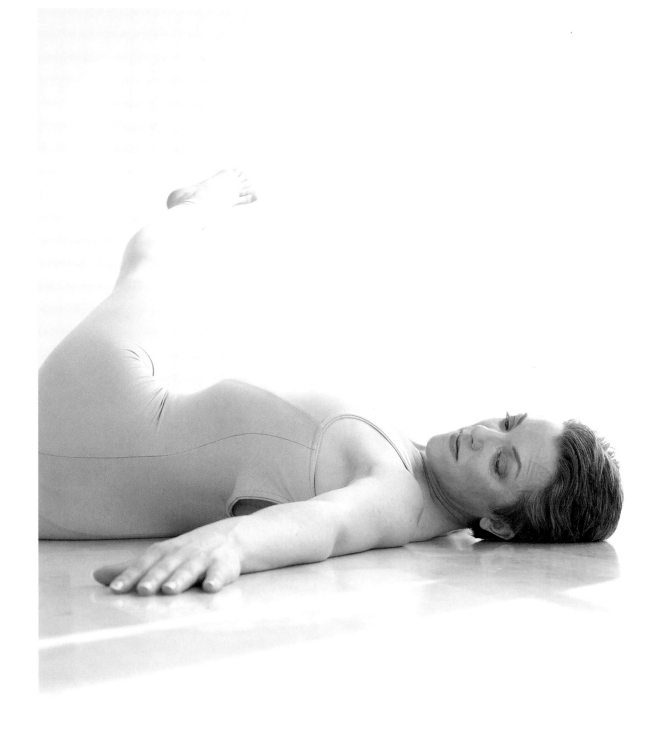

Lying Twist Pose
Jatara Parivartanasana

27

FEW MOVEMENTS provide a release for the spine like gentle twists, such as Lying Twist Pose (Jatara Parivartanasana). The pose feels like it untwists you from the twisted positions that you sometimes unconsciously assume in your daily life. All levels of students enjoy this pose.

SEQUENCING. Most students enjoy this pose at the end of their practice as a transition into relaxation or meditation. But it also can be practiced earlier in your practice if you are feeling fatigued or your lower back is stiff or tight, such as after a long airplane flight.

BENEFITS. Lying Twist Pose stretches the muscles of the lower back, the waist, the rib cage, and the front chest. As such, it can help to facilitate easier breathing, and may have some gentle stimulating effect on the abdominal organs.

CAUTIONS. Proceed carefully if you have diagnosed disc disease in your lower back. Do not practice the variation called Lying Twist Pose on a Stack of Blankets (Figure 27.3) after the first trimester of pregnancy; if you have a hiatal hernia, a detached retina, or glaucoma; or if you are menstruating. Check with your health care professional if you have any concern about elevating your body in this variation.

The Essential Pose *(Figure 27.1)*

PROP: 1 nonskid mat

Spread your mat on a firm and level surface, and lie down with your legs straight out, feet and knees together, arms by your sides, and palms up. Exhale and bend first your right knee and then your left knee, about halfway toward your chest. Inhale, and as you exhale, drop your knees to the right side so that they rest on the floor. Your thighs and lower legs will form a right angle. Make sure that you are resting on your outer right hip, so that your belly button is pointing toward the floor and not the ceiling.

Move your left arm over your head and out in a diagonal line, so that your upper arm stretches past and near your left ear and your left hand rests on the floor. Remember, your left arm should be stretching over your head and not out to the side at shoulder height.

Your right arm is out to the side and at shoulder height. In Lying Twist Pose, you create the stretch by pressing your legs to the right as you stretch through your left arm and turn your belly to the left. It is fine if your left shoulder does not touch the floor. Lift your chest up to create a slight backbend in your upper back. You may enjoy turning your head in the opposite direction of your legs, but it is fine if you keep looking straight up toward the ceiling.

FIGURE 27.1

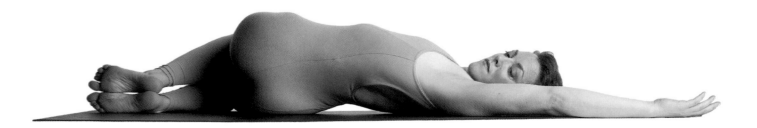

Hold this pose for five to ten breaths. To practice on the other side, roll onto your back and, with an exhalation, lower your feet to the floor. Take a couple of breaths, and repeat to the other side, this time lifting the left knee first. To come out, place both feet on the floor, knees bent, and breathe a breath or two before rolling onto your side and sitting up.

Exploration. There is a simple way to increase the effects on the abdomen. Come into the pose and place your right hand on your right thigh, just above the knee. Your left arm is in a diagonal stretch past and near your left ear. As you exhale, gently press your right leg down and away from you, which will give you more stabilization to increase the twist. Exhale again and press down on your leg and turn your belly strongly to the left. Actively press your left shoulder blade toward the floor. Keep breathing. Stay in the pose for several breaths, release, and repeat to the other side.

Variations

Props: 1 nonskid mat   ✦   2 or 3 blankets

Lying Twist Pose with Your Feet Wide Apart *(Figure 27.2)*. Lie on your mat with your legs straight out, feet and knees together, and arms out by your sides, palms up. Place your feet on the edge of your mat, so that they are parallel to that edge and your knees are wide apart.

As you exhale, drop your knees to the right. Rest your left knee on the inside arch of your right foot. Place your arms out to the sides and on the floor, so that your arms are at shoulder height, palms down. Take several breaths before lifting your knees with an inhalation, and dropping them to the opposite side with an exhalation.

FIGURE 27.2

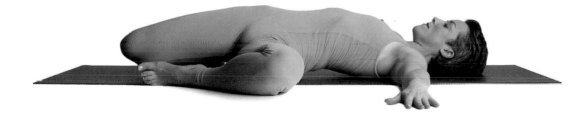

LYING TWIST POSE ON A STACK OF BLANKETS *(Figure 27.3). Refer to the cautions before proceeding.* If you are able to practice this variation, then stack three folded blankets. Remember to lie over the firm, even sides of the folds rather than over the looser ends.

Sit on your props and lie back carefully, so that your shoulders lightly touch the floor, your pelvis is on the props, your knees are bent, and your feet are on the floor. Rotate your knees to the side. Take several gentle breaths and assess your comfort level. Your chest should be open, but your lower back should not be complaining. If you feel that you are too high or if you experience lower back discomfort, then wiggle off the blankets in the direction of your head, roll to your side, and use your hands to help you get up. Lower the height of your props and begin again.

When you are in position, come into the pose. Press your sitting bones down as if you were sitting on a chair. Arch your lower back slightly and lift your chest. The action will open your chest and belly, and give you a pleasant stretch in your outer, top hip.

Hold this stretch for five to ten breaths. Then roll onto your back once again, and lower your feet to the floor. Take a couple of breaths and repeat to the other side, this time lifting the left knee first. To come out of the pose, slide off the blankets in the direction of your head, so that your lower back is supported on the floor. Take one or two breaths, and then roll onto your side before getting up.

FIGURE 27.3

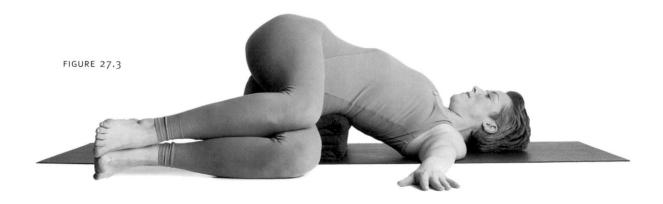

ESPECIALLY FOR TEACHERS

PRIMARY FOCUS. Notice what happens in the middle of your student's body as he twists. When learning this pose, most students twist their legs but not their torsos. Encourage your student to twist so that his belly button points toward the floor. When this happens, he will be resting on the outside of the right hipbone. He may even feel that bone pressing into the floor. If this amount of twist occurs, then the back pelvis and sacrum will be vertical. When this position is established, the twist will be deeper and more effective when the student rolls his shoulder in the opposite direction. But encourage your student to keep his pelvis in this alignment and not to roll back with the belly.

PRIMARY ADJUSTMENT. This adjustment will increase the twist in the belly, which is the core of the body. Ask your student to practice the basic pose to the right. Begin by getting your student's permission both to stand over and to touch him. Bend your knees, keeping a slight arch in your back. Reach around with your right hand, and place it on the back of your student's waist. As you both exhale, use your hand to draw the flesh firmly toward the right, and then to twist it slightly toward the ceiling. The waist is more in contact with the floor, and the right hipbone may press lightly into the floor. Ask your student to take a few breaths before coming out of the pose and practicing to the other side.

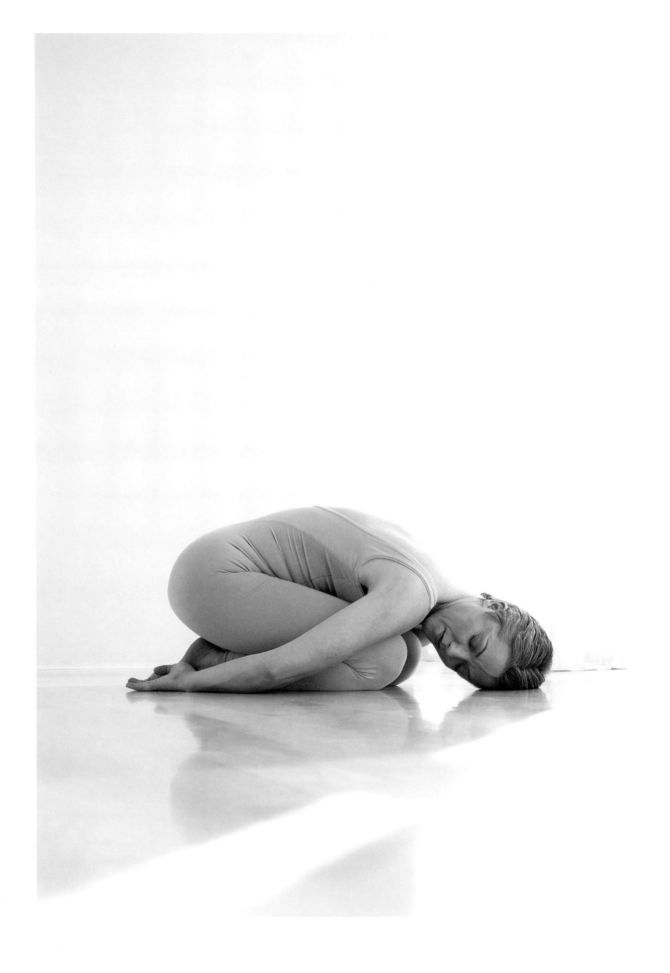

Child's Pose
Adho Mukha Virasana

28

As its name suggests, Child's Pose (Adho Mukha Virasana) resembles the position in which young children so often sleep: the knees are tucked under the tummy, the back is supported by the legs, and the head is gently turned. This pose generates feelings of comfort and release.

Sequencing. Child's Pose can relieve your back after forward bends. You can also use it to transition from the strenuous practice of standing poses and backbends to a time to quiet and calm at the end of your practice.

Benefits. This pose stretches the lower back muscles, quiets the abdominal organs, and enhances introspection. Some women find that it helps to relieve menstrual cramps.

Cautions. Practice this pose with care if you have chronic problems with your knees or pain in your knees. Some students with diagnosed lumbar disc disease may find that Child's Pose exacerbates their symptoms. If this is the case, then do not practice this pose. If you are pregnant, separate your knees to increase comfort when bending forward.

The Essential Pose *(Figure 28.1)*

PROPS: 1 nonskid mat

Place your mat on a firm and level surface, and sit on your heels. Separate your knees approximately 1 foot apart. Exhale, lean forward, and rest your torso on your thighs. Most students enjoy practicing with their arms resting behind them and alongside their legs, their palms facing up, and their shoulders gently rolled forward.

Turn your head to one side, and rest on your cheek. Turn your head in the other direction midway through your practice, so that you spend equal time resting on each cheek. Close your eyes and breathe quietly.

Hold this pose for one to two minutes. To come up, place your hands underneath your shoulders, and push up with an inhalation. Sit on your heels again. Come out of this position by sitting to one side of your feet. Alternatively, come onto your hands and knees, and turn your toes under. Then walk your hands back so that the weight of your body is on your feet and stand up.

EXPLORATION. You can deepen your experience of Child's Pose by paying attention to your breath. Normally, most people are aware of the breath in the front of the body, but rarely in the backs. Because the front ribs are pressed against the thighs or a prop in Child's Pose, the sensation of the movement of the breath is enhanced in the back. Once you are in the pose, slowly inhale and exhale. Notice what happens in your lower back and back waist as you do. Then pay attention to the inner quietness that your breath has helped to create.

VARIATIONS

PROPS: 1 nonskid mat   ✦   1 or more blankets   ✦   1 bolster   ✦   1 face cloth

CHILD'S POSE WITH A BLANKET ON YOUR HEELS *(Figure 28.2)*. Come into the pose. If it feels difficult or uncomfortable, then come up and place one or more blankets in the bend between your heels and your

FIGURE 28.1

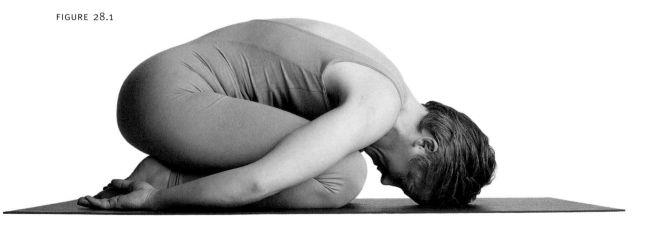

thighs. Fold your blankets in half or in thirds to provide the necessary height. Once you have found the support that you need, continue with the pose. For comfort, rest the side of your face on a face cloth.

CHILD'S POSE WITH SUPPORT *(Figure 28.3)*. Before coming forward, place a bolster between your knees. Then lean forward and rest on the support. Hug the bolster, placing your hands and forearms under it. Alternatively, place your arms along the sides of your body.

ESPECIALLY FOR TEACHERS

PROPS: 1 or more blankets

PRIMARY FOCUS. The most important focus is the comfort of your student's knees. If he or she complains of knee pain, then add one or more folded blankets, as suggested in the first variation, Child's Pose with a Blanket on Your Heels (Figure 28.2). Some students like to place the blanket to fill the hollow at the backs of the knees. In addition, suggest that your student move the knees further apart to increase comfort.

PRIMARY ADJUSTMENT. When your student is comfortable in Child's Pose, stand behind him or her. Ask for and receive permission to touch your student. Then place your palms on the student's outer sacrum, with your fingers pointing diagonally out and back toward you. Press down and back to help lengthen the lower back and stabilize the sacrum. Hold this adjustment for five to seven breaths. This is especially pleasant for a woman during her menstrual period, and it can help to alleviate cramps.

FIGURE 28.2

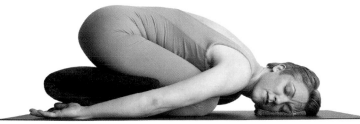

FIGURE 28.3

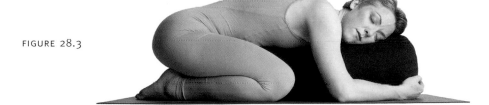

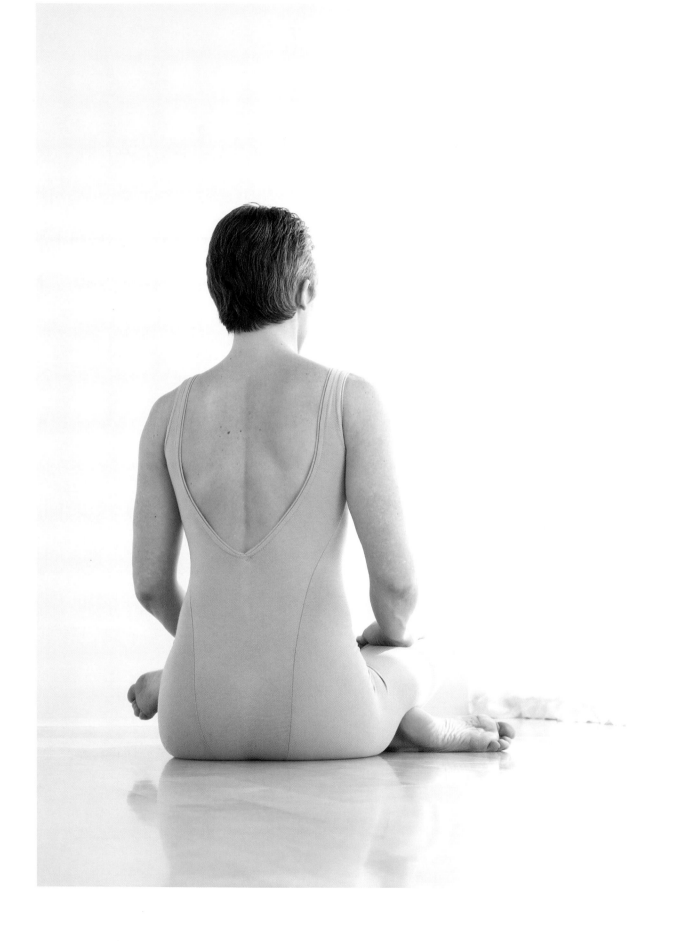

Basic Meditation Pose
Siddhasana

29

FINDING A COMFORTABLE SITTING POSITION is one of the biggest obstacles to beginning a meditation practice. Basic Meditation Pose (Siddhasana) can help to solve that problem. Even if you do not meditate, this pose can give you an understanding of how to sit easily on the floor.

SEQUENCING. Practice this pose by itself for formal meditation. Use at the end of your asana practice, either before or after Basic Relaxation Pose (Figure 30.1), to center and quiet yourself.

BENEFITS. Basic Meditation Pose stretches the adductors and allows your pelvis to be positioned vertically for a comfortable sitting position.

CAUTION. Practice this pose carefully if you have any knee problems.

The Essential Pose *(Figure 29.1)*

PROPS: 1 nonskid mat   ✦   2 or 3 blankets

Spread your mat on a firm and level surface. Sit on your mat and cross your legs in front of you. Each foot helps to support the outside of the opposite thigh. To lift your spine, roll your pubic bone down toward the floor. Make sure that you do not lift your spine by pushing your rib cage forward or by arching your back. Eventually, these two actions would make the pose uncomfortable. Rest the sides of your hands on your thighs lightly. Look straight ahead and then drop your chin slightly, so that your gaze falls about 3 feet in front of you on the floor. You can practice with your eyes open or closed, whichever you prefer. Breathe normally.

After several minutes, change the cross of your legs, putting the opposite leg in front. If you are using this pose for meditation, then alternate the cross of your legs every day. To come out of the pose, simply uncross your legs.

FIGURE 29.1

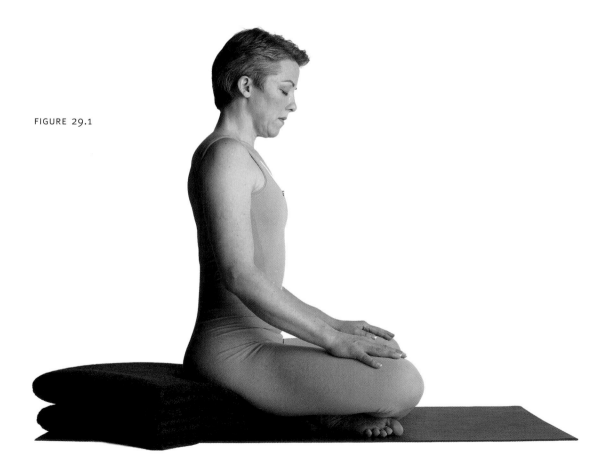

EXPLORATION. Stack two or three folded blankets, and place them at an angle to your mat. Now sit on the corners of the blankets, not on the long edge. When you sit on the corners, your pelvis is supported by the blankets, but your thighs are not in contact with them. This arrangement of the blankets will probably make your pose much more comfortable.

VARIATIONS

PROPS: 1 nonskid mat   ✦   2 or 3 blankets   ✦   1 chair

HALF-LOTUS POSE *(Figure 29.2)*. In Sanskrit, this pose is called Ardha Padmasana. It is a version of Padmasana, or Lotus Pose, and is a good way to learn how to sit cross-legged on the floor.

When you are in Basic Meditation Pose, use your hands to pick up your right leg and simultaneously turn the toes of your right foot strongly toward your right shin. With your foot locked into this position, bring your foot across your body and place it on the opposite thigh, as near to the top as you can. Your heel should now be resting on the top of your thigh. Be sure to reverse which leg is on top midway through the pose. To come out of the pose, simply uncross your legs.

FIGURE 29.2

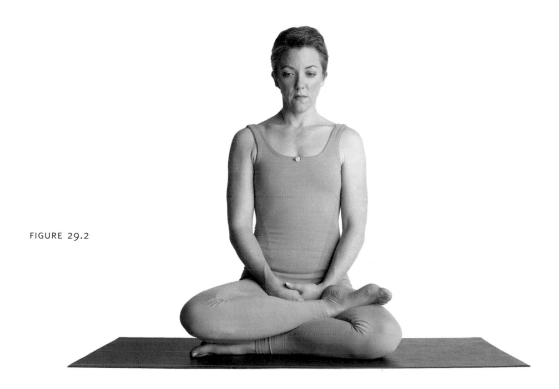

BASIC MEDITATION POSE, SITTING ON A CHAIR *(Figure 29.3)*. Use a chair that has a straight back and no arms. Sit well back in the chair, so that your lower back is completely supported. (If your feet do not reach the floor, then support them with folded blankets.) Separate your feet at an easy distance. Lightly rest your arms on the tops of your thighs or gently clasp the hands as shown. Be sure to change the clasp of your hands midway through the pose. After sitting quietly for twenty to fifty gentle breaths, resume your practice or start the rest of your day.

BASIC MEDITATION POSE WITH ONE LEG ALMOST STRAIGHT *(Figure 29.4)*. This variation is a great way to sit in an almost-cross-legged position if sitting in Basic Meditation Pose causes knee discomfort. Sit on the corner of a stack of blankets, as described in "Exploration" for the Essential Pose. If you experience discomfort in the knee of your top leg, then extend it until it is almost straight, while keeping the bottom leg bent. When your knee becomes healthier, you can try the position with both knees crossed. If extending your top leg does not immediately relieve your discomfort, then practice Basic Meditation Pose, Sitting on a Chair (Figure 29.3).

ESPECIALLY FOR TEACHERS

PRIMARY FOCUS. The primary focus in Basic Meditation Pose is maintaining the natural curves of the spine. When you sit in this way, the vertebral column efficiently supports the weight of the torso. Almost everyone slumps to some degree, whether sitting at a desk, or in a car, or in this pose. Encourage your stu-

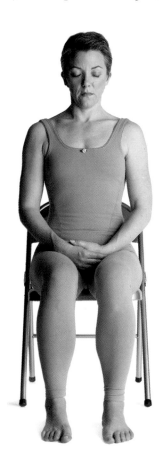

dent to explore what it means to keep the lower lumbar curve. This curve is at the base of the spine, and it creates and sustains the curves in the parts above it.

Most students, even experienced ones, find it useful (if not necessary) to sit on folded blankets to maintain the lumbar curve. If your students are reluctant to use the blankets, then remind them that Zen monks use *zafus* (meditation cushions)—and they are professional sitters! Teaching your students how to sit well will not only help them in this pose, but will provide them with a life skill that can help to prevent lower back problems.

FIGURE 29.3

PRIMARY ADJUSTMENT. To help your student's knees feel more comfortable, try these adjustments. The first is a self-adjustment. Ask your student to bend a knee slightly. Have your student feel behind this knee with the index and middle finger of one hand for the ropelike tendons. When she has located these hamstring tendons, which are called the semimembranosus muscle and the semitendinosus muscle, then ask your student to move her fingers inward until she reaches the hollow at the back of her knee. Have her lay the flat of one palm against her inner calf and thigh evenly, and hold the inner thigh muscles and calf muscles above and below her knee.

Then have your student pull the flesh toward her as she bends her knee the whole way. This adjustment will give her a sense of space behind her knee. Just as your student finishes bending her knee, have her slip her hand out, encouraging even more movement of the flesh toward her. Many students find that this adjustment relieves minor discomfort for bent knees. I recommend this self-adjustment to my students for all bent-knee sitting poses, even if their knees do not hurt, because I believe that it can prevent discomfort. When the adjustment is complete on one side, be sure to have your student practice on the other side.

It is also possible for you, the teacher, to create this adjustment for your student. To begin, ask for and receive permission to touch your student. Then sit on the outside of the leg to be adjusted, and face the student's feet. Reach behind your student's knee as she bends it, and pull outward on the flesh of the inner knee. Be sure to slip your hand out just before your student finishes the movement. This should help her understand the adjustment and its power to relieve minor knee discomfort.

FIGURE 29.4

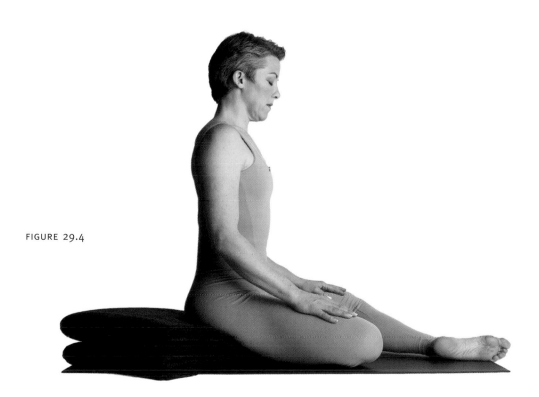

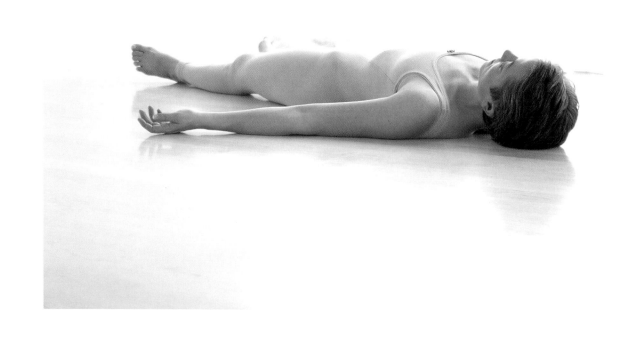

Basic Relaxation Pose and Essential Breathing Practices

Savasana and Pranayama

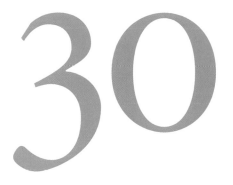

THE PRACTICE OF BASIC RELAXATION POSE (Savasana) is simply one of the healthiest things that you can do for yourself. Learning to relax and breathe well will help you to stay centered in the midst of days filled with multiple commitments—and will help you to recover from nights when you had less sleep than you need.

In 2001, scientist Peter Axt, a professor at a college in Fulda, Germany, told the magazine *Bunte,* "People who prefer lazing in a hammock instead of running the marathon or who take a nap in the middle of the day instead of playing squash have a better chance of living into old age." To antidote stress, especially that caused by work, he advises, "Waste half your free time. Just enjoy lazing around."[1] Ah, another case of modern science catching up with the wisdom of yoga!

SEQUENCING. *Practice Basic Relaxation Pose at the end of your yoga session without fail.* To cure fatigue and jet lag, and to recreate your natural state of balance, you can practice the pose by itself at any other time in the day.

BENEFITS. Basic Relaxation Pose measurably restores all the indices of stress to a healthful balance, including blood pressure, respiratory rate, and brain waves. It allows for an increase in parasympathetic tone in the nervous system, thus facilitating better digestion and assimilation of food, improving fertility, and speeding healing. In addition, studies show improved immune system function when a person regularly practices relaxation. Professor Leslie Walker, director of the Institute of Rehabilitation and Oncology Health at the University of Hull, in Northern England, reported, "Our results show that relaxation and guided imagery can bring about measurable changes in the body's own immunological defenses."[2]

CAUTIONS. If you are pregnant, then practice Side-Lying Relaxation Pose (Figure 30.4). If you have a cold or difficulty breathing easily, then practice Reclining Supported Relaxation Pose (Figure 30.5).

---

1. "Relaxation Techniques Help Cancer Patients—Study," Reuters Limited, 15 April 2000.

2. "Relax! Laziness Is Good for You, Scientist Finds," Reuters Limited, 18 April 2001.

The Essential Pose *(Figure 30.1)*

PROPS: 1 nonskid mat   ✦   1 or 2 blankets
1 bolster   ✦   1 towel   ✦   1 eye cover

To begin Basic Relaxation Pose *and* its variations, do four things first. First, select a quiet, carpeted space. (If you do not have a carpeted space, then use your mat). Second, remove your watch and glasses, loosen your belt buckle, and unbutton clothing that is fitted at your waist. Next, have an eye cover nearby. Finally, if you plan to stay in the pose for ten minutes or longer, or if you tend to get chilly, then plan to cover up with a blanket.

Place a bolster on your mat, and position a rolled towel parallel to, and just beyond, one end of the bolster. Place a folded blanket at the other end of the mat. Sit down, rest your legs over the bolster, and rest your ankles and heels over the towel roll. Carefully lie back. Place your head and neck on the blanket. Draw an imaginary line from your nose to between your feet. Make sure that your legs and arms are equidistant from that line, with your legs gently parted and your feet naturally rolling out. Place the eye cover over your eyes so that the eye cover does not interfere with your nose or breathing.

Position your arms out to the sides so that each is equidistant from your body. Bring your attention to the comfort of your shoulder blades. They are curved bones, so spend a couple of minutes placing them on the flat surface of the floor. In Basic Relaxation Pose, you should feel at ease and supported. If you do not, then adjust yourself so that you do.

Take slow and soft breaths, as your jaw loosens and your body relaxes into the floor. Then release the breath to its own rhythm, but remain aware of it. Notice the tendency of your mind to jump around, especially to the future, such as to all the tasks that you have assigned yourself. When your mind does this, gently bring your attention back to the sensations associated with your breath. Do this time and again. At some point, you may feel quiet enough to observe your breath for a couple of cycles without your mind running away.

FIGURE 30.1

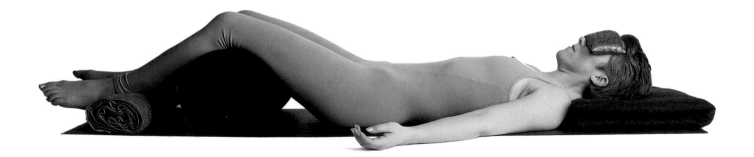

Remain in the pose for five to twenty minutes. To come out, bend one knee, roll to your side, and lie there for a few moments. Use your arms to help you get up slowly. Carry on with the rest of your day slowly and easily.

EXPLORATION. To deepen your experience of Basic Relaxation Pose, pay attention to those muscles that feel especially tense, or focus on a part of your body that is not functioning as well as it should. For example, concentrate on your lower back if that is an area of chronic discomfort, or choose an organ that is involved in a disease process. As previously cited, research shows that the combined techniques of relaxation and visualization can affect immune system function positively. One way to use these techniques is to imagine that each inhalation fills this area with health and well-being, and that each exhalation relaxes it.

VARIATIONS

PROPS: 1 nonskid mat ✦ 6 or more blankets ✦ 1 bolster ✦ 3 or 4 bath towels
          1 chair ✦ 1 to 2 face cloths ✦ 1 block ✦ 1 eye cover

PROP NOTE: Standard Fold Blanket. Fold your blankets to measure 1 inch x 21 inches by 28 inches. This is what I call the standard fold blanket. You will fold or roll standard fold blankets for the following variations and for the breathing practices.

BASIC RELAXATION POSE WITH BACK SUPPORT *(Figure 30.2)*. This variation is particularly suited for use with the breathing practices that come after Basic Relaxation Pose and its variations.

FIGURE 30.2

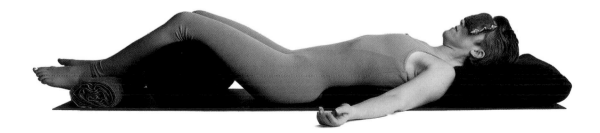

Roll the towel, and fold the blankets into the standard fold, as described in the prop note. From here, fold blanket number one in half the long way. Place this blanket on your mat so that the long edge is parallel to the long sides of the mat. Fold blanket number two in half the short way, and place it *on top of* one end of blanket number one. Sit on the floor at the end of blanket number one so that you are both in contact with the floor and gently pressing against the blanket with your buttocks.

Rest your legs over the bolster, and allow your ankles and heels to rest on the towel roll. Lie back. Make sure that you are completely comfortable and that your back feels fully supported. Position your eye cover on your eyes. Place your arms out to the sides of your body. Because this variation slightly elevates your chest, it will open the lungs and facilitate breathing. In fact, this is an excellent pose to use for your breathing practices.

Remain in this position for five to twenty minutes. When you are ready to come out, do so by stages. Carefully bend one knee at a time, and then roll to your side. Notice all the muscles that contract to help you do this. Don't worry if your eye covering falls off. Now stay on your side for several breaths, and then gradually open your eyes. Use your arms to help you sit up slowly. Take one more gentle, long breath before standing up carefully.

RELAXATION POSE WITH YOUR LEGS ON A CHAIR *(Figure 30.3)*. In addition to imparting all the benefits of Basic Relaxation Pose, this variation is particularly helpful for those with lower back pain.

Place your chair in the center of the room. (If you are practicing with a mat, then do *not* place the chair legs on it, because they can puncture or tear the mat.) Fold a standard fold blanket in half the short way to place under your head and neck. Place a folded towel on the chair seat for your Achilles tendons.

Sit down with your knees bent and your feet pointed toward the chair seat. Lie back and place the blanket under your head and neck. Bend your knees toward your chest, and then place your lower legs on the chair seat. Position your legs on the towel. Take a moment to make sure that the height of the chair is correct for you. If it is, then your lower back will feel supported, your lower legs will rest comfortably on the seat, and your heels will not be lifted off of it. If your heels are lifted, then the chair is too high for you.

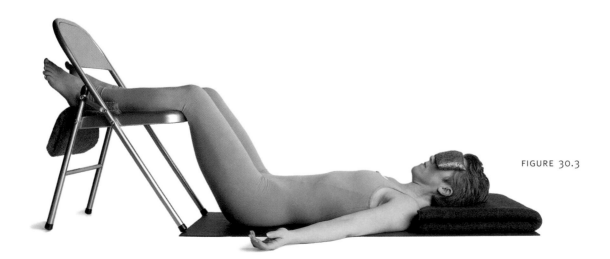

FIGURE 30.3

You can remedy this either by using a lower chair or by elevating your torso. To do so, lie on a few stacked standard fold blankets that you have folded in half on the long side.

Adjust the position of the blanket under your head and neck as needed. Make sure that the blanket completely supports your neck.

Stay in the pose for up to twenty minutes. Concentrate on letting your lower back drop down into the floor, and release any tension that may have accumulated there. During this relaxation, be sure to take at least ten long, slow breaths. When your relaxation is over, roll carefully to your side and sit up slowly. Take care not to bump yourself on the chair as you do so.

SIDE-LYING RELAXATION POSE *(Figure 30.4)*. This variation offers an alternative to those who cannot relax when lying on the back. I strongly recommend that women past the first trimester of pregnancy use this variation as their daily relaxation practice. This is also a great position to assume during the middle stages of labor.

This variation requires three blankets, which start in the standard fold. Blanket number one remains in the standard fold and is for under your torso. Fold blanket number two the short way for use under your head. Fold blanket number three the long way for placement between your lower legs and knees.

Now lie down, on one side, on blanket number one. Place blanket number two under your head, positioned in whatever way feels comfortable to you. Blanket number three goes between your lower legs, so that your top knee and top foot are supported at the same distance from the floor and your shin is parallel to the floor. Rest the back of your bottom hand on one or two face cloths for comfort. Place your eye cover on the side of your neck. Draw the bolster close to your body and drape your top arm over it.

You can remain in Side-Lying Relaxation Pose for up to twenty minutes. To deepen your enjoyment, make sure that all your props are placed exactly as you want them. You will feel as if you could go to sleep, but don't. Remember to take a few deep breaths as you start the practice. This will help you be able to relax without falling asleep. When you are finished with the pose, slowly get up by using your arms for support.

FIGURE 30.4

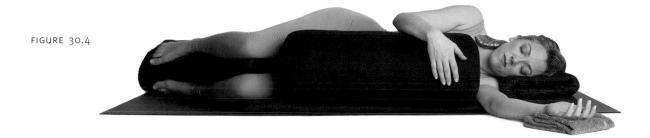

Reclining Supported Relaxation Pose *(Figure 30.5)*. You will enjoy this variation as a change from lying flat. Pregnant and menstruating women love the deep sense of well-being that it engenders. This variation can also be soothing if you have a cold or other respiratory problems. It is a pleasant one to use with any of the essential breathing practices.

You will need one mat, one block, one bolster, three blankets, one towel, one face cloth, and one eye cover. It takes effort to fold, position, and adjust the props, so think of doing so as taking a vacation. Although it takes planning to get there, when you finally arrive you are glad that you did it all!

Fold the blankets into the standard fold. Then fold blankets number one and number two in half the short way. Roll blanket number three from the short side. Roll the towel for placement under your Achilles tendons, and fold the face cloth for placement under your head and neck.

Spread your mat on the floor, and position the block at one end. Place the bolster on the diagonal, with one end supported by the block. Sit in front of the bolster, with your hips touching it. Place the blanket roll under your knees and the towel roll under your Achilles tendons. Lie back.

Place the folded face cloth under your head and neck. Position blankets number one and number two for your forearms. Place your eye cover over your eyes, and rest your forearms on the blankets.

If you experience any lower back pain, then elevate yourself by adding folded blankets on top of the bolster, so that you are at an angle that is higher than 45 degrees.

Relax your jaw and feel your body supported by the props and the floor. A simple and effective focusing technique is to breathe slowly and softly, inhaling to the count of 10, exhaling, and then starting again.

To come out of the pose, bend your knees toward your chest and roll to one side. Lie there for a moment, and then use the support of your arms to get up.

Especially for Teachers

Primary Focus. Despite its many benefits, many yoga students—and even yoga teachers—do not make time to incorporate Basic Relaxation Pose into their daily lives.

FIGURE 30.5

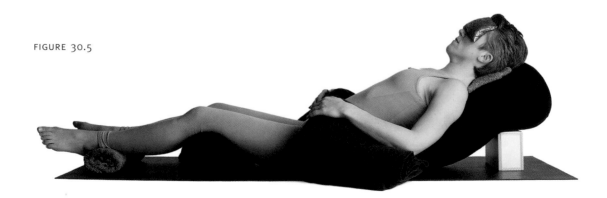

I used to notice a thought that stopped me from practicing Basic Relaxation Pose at the end of my yoga session or at some other time during the day: *If I lie down to relax, then I will never get up.* I worried that I might lie there for three hours and not accomplish what I would like. For me, using a timer is a liberating strategy: I have the confidence that I will have a chance to make a clear decision about whether to stay in the pose or get up at the end of twenty minutes. Using the timer to create a boundary frees me to let go and enjoy the relaxation.

PRIMARY ADJUSTMENT. The student's head position is critical to relaxation. Make sure that your student places his head so that the forehead is slightly higher than the chin. It is akin to bowing the head for meditation or prayer, and it serves to quiet the nervous system.

Here is a simple adjustment. When your student is lying in Basic Relaxation Pose, sit by his head. Ask for and receive your student's permission to touch him. Reach your hands under the back of his neck, so that your thumbs are along the jaw. Slide your hands toward yourself, so that you support the lowest part of the back of the skull. Continue this movement: your hands are now rolling the head toward you and then the chin down. This is done is one smooth movement. It is not necessary to lift the student's head very high up off the floor. To hone your skills, practice this adjustment with a friend or family member until it feels natural and easy.

ESSENTIAL BREATHING PRACTICES

Just as the yoga tradition offers you the opportunity to move with attention, so, too, it offers you the chance to breathe with awareness. Asana is to physical exercise what pranayama is to breathing technique. These simple, effective techniques help you to relax, to center, and to slow down. Try to practice one every day for four months. To cycle through them will take one year. By that time, you will be well established in breathing practice.

RECOMMENDATIONS FOR BREATHING PRACTICES. The points that follow are intended to give you a safe and satisfying experience of the breathing practices.

✦ The three practices that I have selected can be done by almost anyone. If you are unsure about whether all are suitable for you, then just do Breathing Practice #1: Even Inhalation, Even Exhalation.

✦ These practices naturally fit at the beginning of Basic Relaxation Pose or some of its variations. They allow you to relax your body and to be better able to focus on your breath.

✦ Practice for five minutes at the beginning of your relaxation.

✦ Keep your eyes closed throughout practice.

✦ Stay completely relaxed: do not tense your face, your hands, or your belly.

✦ Initiate your inhalations by lifting your ribs out and by allowing your lungs and abdomen to expand naturally. Do *not* begin the breath by pushing out or bulging out your abdomen. There are no lungs here: you will just weaken your abdominal wall by breathing in this manner.

✦ To aid concentration, let your breath make a soft sound by slightly restricting the back of your throat. This noise should be audible only to you.

✦ Applicable cautions are listed at the beginning of a breathing practice.

BREATHING PRACTICE #1:
EVEN INHALATION, EVEN EXHALATION
SAMA VRTTI

Set yourself up in Basic Relaxation Pose with Back Support (Figure 30.2) or in Reclining Supported Relaxation Pose (Figure 30.5). When comfortably established in the pose, begin with slow, soft breaths. With each inhalation, gradually increase the length of the breath. Follow it with an equal exhalation.

Try to keep your inhalations and exhalations even. About every second round, just breathe normally, and then return to the longer breaths. *Do not force the breath:* just concentrate on the evenness and smoothness of each one. Think of balancing what you take in with what you give out. This is the dance of the breath, the dance of life, that keeps you in balance.

Try this breathing practice for three to five minutes and then let your breath return to normal. Continue to pay attention to what the breath does on its own. After you have concluded Breathing Practice #1: Even Inhalation, Even Exhalation, let Basic Relaxation Pose with Back Support or Reclining Supported Relaxation Pose naturally follow. Consider focusing on a part of your body that is not functioning as it should. Imagine that your exhalation relaxes that area, and that your next inhalation fills it with health and well-being.

When you are finished, roll gently to your side, lie there for a few breaths, and then use your arms to help you sit up.

BREATHING PRACTICE #2:
LONG INHALATION, SHORT EXHALATION
VISAMA VRTTI I

Do not attempt this breathing practice if you have high blood pressure or are pregnant. Set yourself up in Basic Relaxation Pose with Back Support (Figure 30.2) or in Reclining Supported Relaxation Pose (Figure 30.5). When you are comfortably established in the pose, begin with slow, soft breaths. With each inhalation, gradually increase the length of the breath. Follow it with an equal exhalation.

The emphasis here is on increasing your inhalation until it is two times longer than your exhalation. But don't force this ratio. At every second round, take a normal inhalation and exhalation, and then return to the rhythm of longer inhalations.

I cannot say it often enough: Do not force the breath. Just concentrate on the evenness and smoothness of each inhalation and each exhalation. Imagine that each inhalation is bringing in energy and life, and that each exhalation is letting go of discomfort.

Practice for three to five minutes, and then let your breath return to normal. Continue to pay attention to what the breath does on its own. Let Basic Relaxation Pose with Back Support or Reclining Supported Relaxation Pose follow naturally. When you are finished, roll easily to your side, lie there for a few breaths, and then use your arms to help you sit up.

BREATHING PRACTICE #3:
SHORT INHALATION, LONG EXHALATION
VISAMA VRTTI II

Set yourself up in Basic Relaxation Pose with Back Support (Figure 30.2) or in Supported Reclining Relaxation Pose (Figure 30.5). When you are comfortable, begin to breathe slow and soft breaths. With each inhalation, gradually increase the length of your breath. Follow it with an equal exhalation.

To begin Breathing Practice #3, inhale a normal amount and then elongate your exhalation. Follow this round with a normal inhalation and exhalation. Once again, inhale normally and then elongate your exhalation. Then return to a normal inhalation and exhalation.

At no time should you feel agitated or out of breath. Continue with a normal inhalation and an exhalation that is twice as long. Count each inhalation: *1,001, 1,002, 1,003.* Follow this by counting each exhalation: *1,001, 1,002, 1,003, 1,004, 1,005, 1,006.* Make sure that you follow each longer exhalation with a normal inhalation and exhalation. Keep this rhythm going for up to five minutes. The prolonged exhalation will increase the pressure inside your lungs and help to force open the airways so that the next inhalation is easier. This can be especially helpful for those with asthma.

End with several equal inhalations and exhalations. Then bring your attention to what the breath does on its own. Return to Basic Relaxation Pose with Back Support or Reclining Supported Relaxation Pose. When you are finished, gently roll to your side, lie here for a few breaths, and use your arms to help you sit up.

ESPECIALLY FOR TEACHERS

PRIMARY FOCUS. Teaching students to breathe with awareness is a more subtle art than teaching them to practice asana with awareness. All aspects of the breath are important: the length, the quality, the texture, and the rhythm. But in the beginning, the student should be encouraged to focus almost exclusively on creating evenness in the breath. This evenness facilitates a deep inner calmness in the nervous system. It is this equanimity of the nervous system that provides the necessary foundation for meditative mind.

Sit beside your student. Ask her to make a slight sound with the breath while practicing. Listen to the sound and, when necessary, encourage her to breathe with less force if that is what helps to create and maintain evenness in the breath.

PRIMARY ADJUSTMENT. Pay primary attention to the positioning of the student's chest during the practice. It should be open and yet supported at the same time, so that there can be a free movement of the diaphragm. Some students may enjoy being propped up higher to facilitate easier breathing. Finally, make sure that the student's chin is dropped lower than the forehead to create a quieter state of mind.

PART FOUR

THE PRACTICE

T HE MEASURE OF THE SUCCESS of this book is what happens now. It is my deep hope that you are willing—and even eager—to practice what you read about in the previous pages. This part of the book will guide you as you make getting onto your yoga mat a regular part of your life.

THE SACRED CIRCLE

Whether you practice on your own or in a class, begin each session by creating a sacred circle. You can do this in two parts. First, make the act of physically stepping onto your mat the symbol for creating an atmosphere of safety, focus, and self-exploration. Second, when on the mat, state a practice intention, either silently or aloud. You can repeat this intention several times during your practice.

To help you get started, I suggest practice intentions that I call Mantras for Daily Practice. You will find these with each practice sequence. *Mantra* comes from the Sanskrit words *manas,* which means "mind," and *tra,* or "to transcend." In the *Encyclopedic Dictionary of Yoga,* author Georg Feuerstein writes that a mantra "is thought or intention expressed as sound."[1] In the context of this book, a mantra can help you gain a new perspective on your yoga practice.

Stating your intention is a way to empower yourself. Use the mantras (intentions) in this book, if you wish, or make up your own. Let yourself be guided by a virtue or skill that you would like to cultivate or celebrate. *Remember, yoga practice is not about being perfect: it is about being kind to yourself.* For example, on a day when standing poses are a focus, you may say, "I commit to staying present with my breath as I move." On a busy day you may declare, "I promise to stay on the mat for fifteen minutes and not be distracted by other duties." When you experience resistance to practicing, step on your mat and say, "Right here, right now," which is a Mantra for Daily Living from my second book, *Living Your Yoga: Finding the Spiritual in Everyday Life.*[2] As you work with the practice of setting your intentions throughout the coming days, weeks, and months, notice how kindness affects your practice and your life.

If you are teaching a class, then step onto your mat, and take a moment at the front of the class to silently state your intention for the period. Recall the joy that you feel from your practice and your teaching, and let that be the foundation of all that you say and do as you teach this class. Know that you are guiding yourself and your students within a sacred circle.

Students and teachers, you can end your personal practice or class with your hands in Namaste and with a slight bow. (For an example of Namaste, see Figure 2.3 in Part Three, "The Poses.") As you do, silently restate your intention. Take an extra moment to express your gratitude for having the time and space to devote to yoga. Remembering to be grateful adds richness to the simplest of life's activities.

SEQUENCING AND WHY IT MATTERS

All yoga poses are done in relationship with all others. Therefore, the effect of each pose can be measured, in part, by the pose that came before it and the one that comes after it. For example, if you are focusing on forward bends, then you should practice basic forward bends first and gradually move toward more challenging ones, as your body accommodates the movements necessary to bend forward. Working in this way will not only take you deeper, it will also allow your body to warm up slowly, which will help to prevent injury.

Another principle of sequencing is to practice the poses that encourage systemic effects and involve the large muscles first. For this reason, the sequences suggested in *30 Essential Yoga Poses* generally begin with

---

1. Feuerstein, *Encyclopedic Dictionary of Yoga,* 211.

2. Judith Lasater, Ph.D., P.T., *Living Your Yoga: Finding the Spiritual in Everyday Life* (Berkeley, Calif.: Rodmell Press, 2000), 73.

standing poses, and not with floor work, which requires much smaller movements. As you progress in any given practice period, your body warms up and your mind cools down. The order of the poses both creates and reflects this change.

Finally, an effective sequence of poses never juxtaposes an extreme movement with its opposite extreme movement. For example, the sequences presented here do not suggest a deep backbend followed by a deep forward bend. Instead, after a deep backbend, it is wise to transition with poses that gradually introduce the opposite movement to the body, such as gentle twists. The poses in this book are sequenced with these principles in mind.

PROPS AND WHY THEY MATTER

A prop is an aid that is used to support you when you are not quite able to do the pose, to help you to explore a pose in a new way, or to facilitate ease and relaxation in active and restorative poses.

In *30 Essential Yoga Poses*, props can be grouped into five categories: props you stand on, props you lie on, props you place on your body, props you rest on or against, and other. Here is a list of props, by category, that you will need to practice with this book. Some props will be used in more than one category.

PROPS YOU STAND ON: 2 nonskid mats

PROPS YOU LIE ON: 6 or more blankets ✦ 1 bolster
2 blocks ✦ 2 pillows ✦ 3 or 4 bath towels

PROPS YOU PLACE ON YOUR BODY:
1 eye cover ✦ 2 face cloths ✦ 1 strap

PROPS YOU REST ON OR AGAINST:
1 chair ✦ 1 wall ✦ 1 pole ✦ 1 low bench

OTHER: 1 mirror

TIPS FOR PRACTICE

Take time to prepare for your practice. Here are some simple tips to ensure that it is safe and satisfying:
   ✦ When possible, practice at the same time and in the same place each day.
   ✦ Wait at least three hours after eating before you practice. Some people prefer to wait even longer.
   ✦ You may enjoy a shower before your practice to soothe and relax yourself.
   ✦ Wear loose and comfortable clothes, and have bare feet. Be sure to tie back long hair. Take off your watch.
   ✦ If you are practicing at home, then remove your glasses or contact lenses, especially during poses that are done with the eyes closed, such as Basic Meditation Pose (Figure 29.1), Basic Relaxation Pose (Figure 30.1), and their variations.

✦ If you are practicing at a studio, then you can take a towel to cover the mat. Certainly take your own eye covering, such as an eyebag or face cloth. This is a very personal prop, and using your own will prevent the spread of bacteria. If wool makes your skin itch, then take your own cotton blanket to cover your body under the wool blankets if they are all that is provided.

✦ Practice at your comfort level. Your body is not an enemy to be overcome. Pushing your body too far or too fast can result in injury, as well as contribute to a resistance to practicing the next time.

✦ It is important that you allow at least five minutes for Basic Relaxation Pose (Figure 30.1) or one of its variations at the end of each practice session. This period of relaxation allows your body to rest and integrate the effect of the poses.

✦ Unless indicated otherwise, each practice session is intended to last about one hour. That allows adequate time for Basic Relaxation Pose (Figure 30.1), as well as a well-rounded practice of the active poses.

✦ You may wonder how long you should hold the poses. Let your breath, not the clock, be your timer. Except for Basic Relaxation Pose (Figure 30.1) and its variations, which I suggest that you hold for ten minutes or longer, you can begin by holding the poses for three to five breaths. Gradually, as you learn the pose, you will naturally find it easier to stay longer. The most important thing, however, is the quality of, not the length of, your breath. In other words, if your breath is easy, relaxed, and flowing, then you can probably hold the pose longer with safety and benefit. If your breath is ragged or strained, or if you find yourself holding your breath, then it is better to come out of the pose. Remember to pay attention to your body throughout the pose: coming in, being there, and coming out. Listen to your breath and stay attentive to what it is telling you about staying in the pose.

✦ Honor yourself: Acknowledge your limitations without accepting them as your fate. Remember, practice is about exploring your possibilities. This may begin with becoming aware of your tendency to chase perfection. Letting go of that will aid your practice now and in the years to come.

Four Practice Choices

Developing and maintaining a home practice can be challenging, especially for beginning students. You may wonder, *Where do I begin?* This part of *30 Essential Yoga Poses* offers four approaches to support your personal practice. I call them "Busy Days Practice," "Day-of-the-Week Practice," "Theme Practice," and "The 30 Essential Yoga Poses Practice."

Each session discussion includes the name of the sequence, the purpose of the practice, a brief message for teachers, as well as a Mantra for Daily Practice. The name of each pose appears in English and Sanskrit, and a photograph of the pose is shown. The figure number that accompanies each photograph corresponds to the numbering system in Part Three, "The Poses."

I suggest either the essential pose or a variation. If practicing what I suggest does not feel right for you on a given day, refer to the alternate versions of that pose in Part Three, and select what meets your needs.

Busy Days Practice

Ironically, the days when you most need yoga may be the days when you feel that you have the least amount of time to practice. I designed this sequence to allow you to use a short period of time very effectively. I find it helpful on days when I rise very early to catch a flight, on holidays when family obligations beckon, and when I need to devote many hours to an urgent project.

If your time is so constrained that you cannot fit this fifteen-minute to twenty-minute practice into your day, then I suggest that you commit yourself to doing five minutes of Basic Relaxation Pose (Figure 30.1). You might look on these five minutes as your "minimum daily requirement" of yoga.

PURPOSE: To live the understanding that more is not necessarily better.

A WORD TO TEACHERS: There is no such thing as too little yoga practice.

MANTRA FOR DAILY PRACTICE: There is enough time.

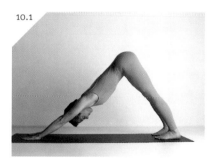

DOWNWARD-FACING DOG POSE
ADHO MUKHA SVANASANA

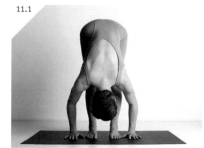

STANDING FORWARD BEND POSE
UTTANASANA

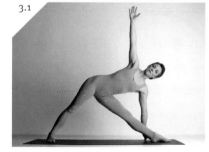

EXTENDED TRIANGLE POSE
UTTHITA TRIKONASANA

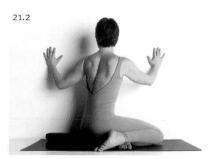

SIMPLE SEATED-TWIST POSE AT THE WALL
BHARADVAJASANA

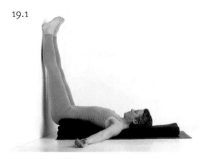

ELEVATED LEGS-UP-THE-WALL POSE
VIPARITA KARANI

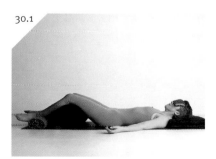

BASIC RELAXATION POSE
SAVASANA

THIS WELL-ROUNDED PRACTICE INCLUDES SOME NEW THINGS AND SOME REPETITION EVERY DAY.

Day One

Day-of-the-Week Practice

PURPOSE: To establish the strength of the legs and the spine.

A WORD TO TEACHERS: Basic standing poses are the foundation of learning how to stand on your own two feet.

MANTRA FOR DAILY PRACTICE: To begin is the victory.

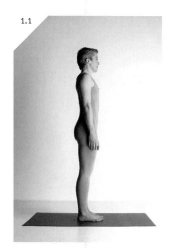

1.1

MOUNTAIN POSE
TADASANA

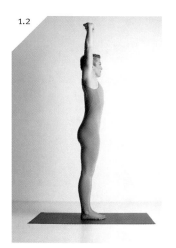

1.2

MOUNTAIN POSE WITH YOUR
ARMS OVERHEAD ~ TADASANA

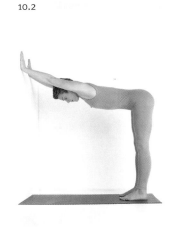

10.2

HALF-DOG POSE AT THE WALL
ADHO MUKHA SVANASANA

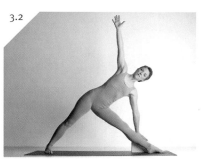

3.2

EXTENDED TRIANGLE POSE WITH YOUR HAND
ON A BLOCK ~ UTTHITA TRIKONASANA

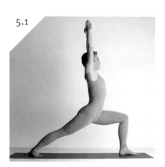

5.1

WARRIOR I POSE
VIRABHADRASANA I

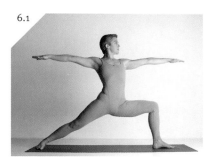

6.1

WARRIOR II POSE
VIRABHADRASANA II

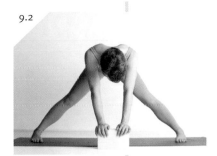

WIDE-LEG STANDING FORWARD BEND POSE
WITH A BLOCK
PRASARITA PADOTTANASANA

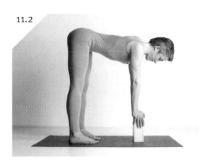

STANDING FORWARD BEND POSE WITH YOUR
HANDS ON A BLOCK ~ UTTANASANA

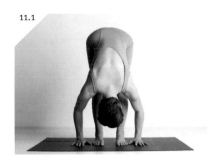

STANDING FORWARD BEND POSE
UTTANASANA

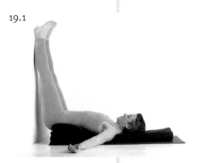

ELEVATED LEGS-UP-THE-WALL POSE
VIPARITA KARANI

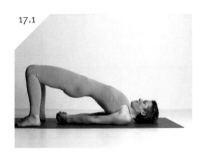

BRIDGE POSE
SETU BANDHASANA

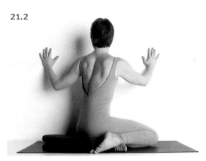

SIMPLE SEATED-TWIST POSE AT THE WALL
BHARADVAJASANA

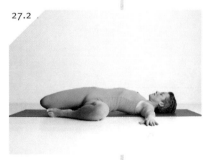

LYING TWIST POSE WITH YOUR FEET WIDE
APART ~ JATARA PARIVARTANASANA

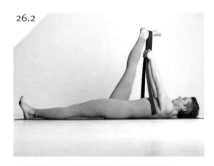

RECLINING LEG-STRETCH POSE WITH A
STRAP ~ SUPTA PADANGUSTHASANA

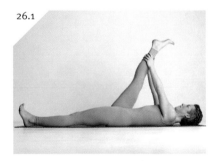

RECLINING LEG-STRETCH POSE
SUPTA PADANGUSTHASANA

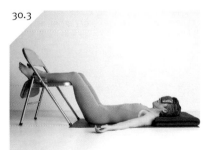

BASIC RELAXATION POSE WITH YOUR
LEGS ON A CHAIR ~ SAVASANA WITH BREATHING PRACTICE #1:
EVEN INHALATION, EVEN EXHALATION ~ SAMA VRTTI

Day Two

PURPOSE: To link the hamstring stretches of standing poses with seated hamstring stretches.

A WORD TO TEACHERS: Remind your students to move from the hip joints and not from the spine in seated poses.

MANTRA FOR DAILY PRACTICE: The opposite of action is not inaction: it is presence.

1.2
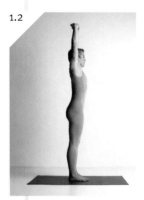
MOUNTAIN POSE WITH YOUR ARMS OVERHEAD ~ TADASANA

2.1
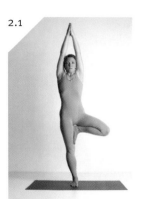
TREE POSE VRKSASANA

2.3
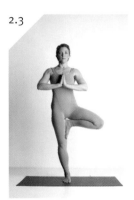
TREE POSE WITH YOUR HANDS IN NAMASTE VRKSASANA

3.5
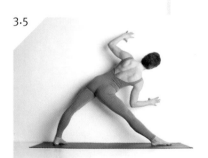
EXTENDED TRIANGLE POSE, FACING THE WALL ~ UTTHITA TRIKONASANA

3.1
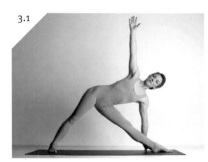
EXTENDED TRIANGLE POSE UTTHITA TRIKONASANA

4.2
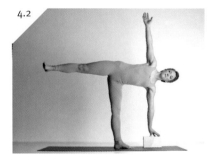
HALF-MOON POSE WITH YOUR HAND ON A BLOCK ~ ARDHA CHANDRASANA

4.1
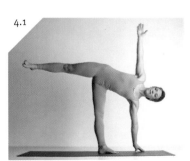
HALF-MOON POSE ARDHA CHANDRASANA

6.2
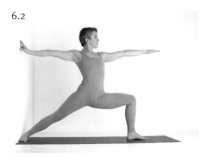
WARRIOR II POSE WITH YOUR BACK FOOT AGAINST THE WALL ~ VIRABHADRASANA II

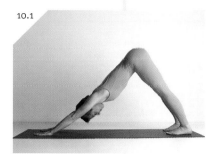

10.1

DOWNWARD-FACING DOG POSE
ADHO MUKHA SVANASANA

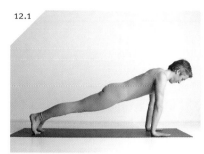

12.1

UP-PLANK POSE
CHATURANGA DANDASANA

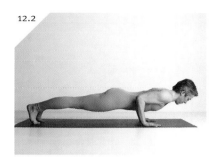

12.2

DOWN-PLANK POSE
CHATURANGA DANDASANA

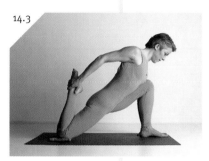

14.3

LUNGE POSE, HOLDING YOUR ANKLE
ANJANEYASANA

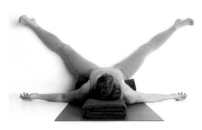

19.3

ELEVATED LEGS-UP-THE-WALL POSE WITH
LEGS IN SEATED-ANGLE POSE
VIPARITA KARANI

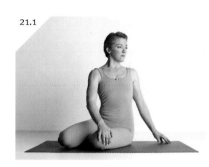

21.1

SIMPLE SEATED-TWIST POSE
BHARADVAJASANA

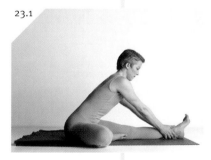

23.1

HEAD-OF-THE-KNEE POSE
JANU SIRSASANA

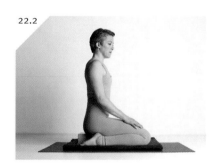

22.2

HERO–HEROINE POSE, SITTING ON A BLOCK
VIRASANA

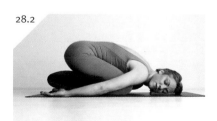

28.2

CHILD'S POSE WITH A BLANKET ON YOUR
HEELS ~ ADHO MUKHA VIRASANA

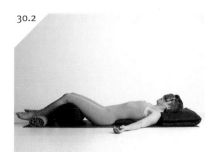

30.2

BASIC RELAXATION POSE WITH BACK SUPPORT ~ SAVASANA
WITH BREATHING PRACTICE #1: EVEN INHALATION, EVEN EXHALATION ~ SAMA VRTTI

Day Three

PURPOSE: Backbends open the lungs and free the heart.

A WORD TO TEACHERS: Healthy backs bend in all directions.

MANTRA FOR DAILY PRACTICE: It's not the letting go that hurts: it's the holding on.

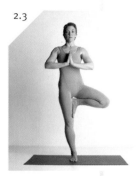

2.3

TREE POSE WITH YOUR
HANDS IN NAMASTE
VRKSASANA

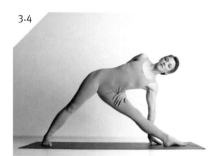

3.4

EXTENDED TRIANGLE POSE WITH YOUR ARM
BEHIND YOUR WAIST
UTTHITA TRIKONASANA

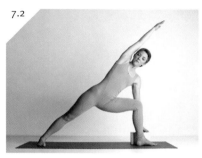

7.2

EXTENDED SIDE-ANGLE STRETCH POSE WITH
YOUR HAND ON A BLOCK
UTTHITA PARSVAKONASANA

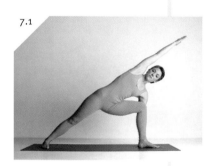

7.1

EXTENDED SIDE-ANGLE STRETCH POSE
UTTHITA PARSVAKONASANA

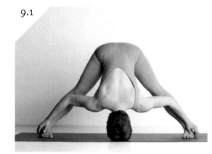

9.1

WIDE-LEG STANDING FORWARD BEND POSE
PRASARITA PADOTTANASANA

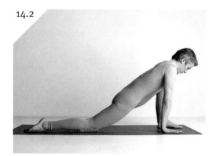

14.2

LUNGE POSE WITH YOUR BACK KNEE DOWN
ANJANEYASANA

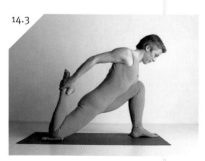

14.3

LUNGE POSE, HOLDING YOUR ANKLE
ANJANEYASANA

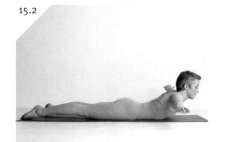

15.2

COBRA POSE WITH YOUR ARMS STRETCHED
TO THE SIDES ~ BHUJANGASANA

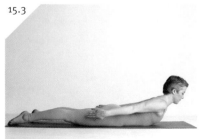

15.3

COBRA POSE WITH YOUR ARMS STRETCHED
BACKWARD ~ BHUJANGASANA

15.4

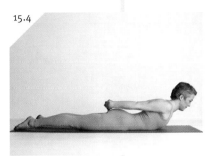

COBRA POSE WITH YOUR HANDS CLASPED
BEHIND YOUR BACK ~ BHUJANGASANA

16.1

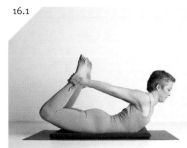

BOW POSE
DHANURASANA

17.1

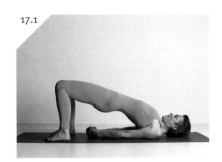

BRIDGE POSE
SETU BANDHASANA

18.2

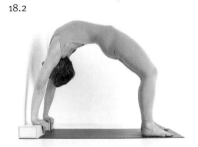

UPWARD-FACING BOW POSE AT THE WALL
AND WITH YOUR HANDS ELEVATED ON
BLOCKS ~ URDHVA DHANURASANA

18.3

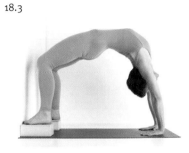

UPWARD-FACING BOW POSE AT THE WALL
AND WITH YOUR FEET ELEVATED ON BLOCKS
URDHVA DHANURASANA

18.1

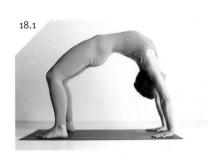

UPWARD-FACING BOW POSE
URDHVA DHANURASANA

20.1

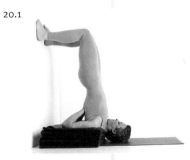

SUPPORTED SHOULDERSTAND POSE
SALAMBA SARVANGASANA

21.1

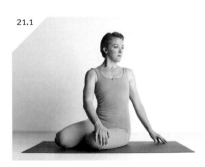

SIMPLE SEATED-TWIST POSE
BHARADVAJASANA

27.3

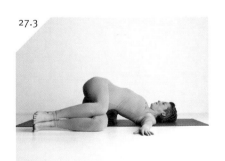

LYING TWIST POSE ON A STACK OF BLANKETS
JATARA PARIVARTANASANA

26.2

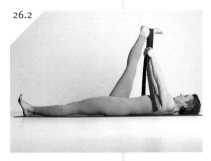

RECLINING LEG-STRETCH POSE WITH A
STRAP ~ SUPTA PADANGUSTHASANA

26.1

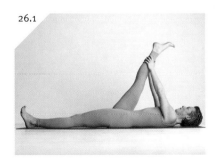

RECLINING LEG-STRETCH POSE
SUPTA PADANGUSTHASANA

30.3

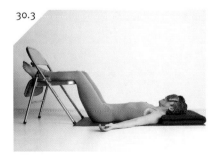

BASIC RELAXATION POSE WITH YOUR LEGS
ON A CHAIR ~ SAVASANA ~ WITH BREATHING
PRACTICE #3: SHORT INHALATION,
LONG EXHALATION ~ VISAMA VRTTI II

Day Four

PURPOSE: To focus on poses that strengthen the arms and create more flexibility in the upper back.

A WORD TO TEACHERS: Strength in the arms saves the back.

MANTRA FOR DAILY PRACTICE: What would my life be like without the thought *I can't*?

3.4

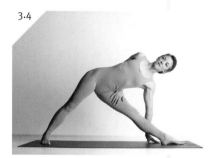

EXTENDED TRIANGLE POSE
WITH YOUR ARM BEHIND YOUR WAIST
UTTHITA TRIKONASANA

6.1

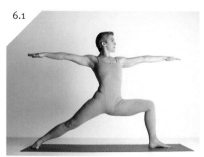

WARRIOR II POSE
VIRABHADRASANA II

8.2

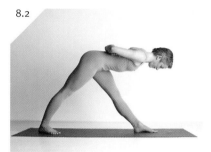

SIDE-CHEST STRETCH POSE, HALFWAY DOWN
PARSVOTTANASANA

8.1

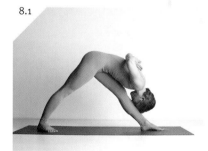

SIDE-CHEST STRETCH POSE
PARSVOTTANASANA

10.3

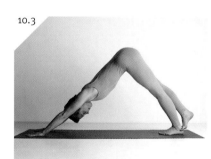

DOWNWARD-FACING DOG POSE WITH THE
TOES OF ONE FOOT ON THE HEEL OF THE
OTHER ~ ADHO MUKHA SVANASANA

13.2

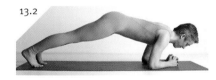

13.3

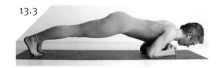

HEADSTAND PREPARATION POSE,
MOVING BACKWARD AND FORWARD
SALAMBA SIRSASANA

13.1

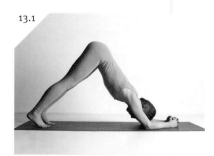

HEADSTAND PREPARATION POSE
SALAMBA SIRSASANA

12.1

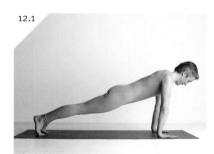

UP-PLANK POSE
CHATURANGA DANDASANA

12.2

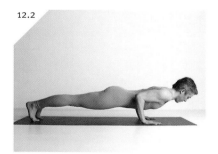

DOWN-PLANK POSE
CHATURANGA DANDASANA

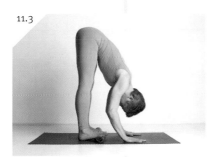

STANDING FORWARD BEND POSE
WITH A ROLLED MAT UNDER YOUR TOES
UTTANASANA

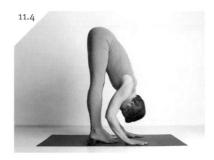

STANDING FORWARD BEND POSE
WITH A ROLLED MAT UNDER YOUR HEELS
UTTANASANA

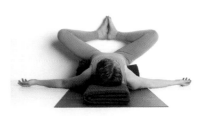

ELEVATED LEGS-UP-THE-WALL POSE
WITH LEGS IN BOUND-ANGLE POSE
VIPARITA KARANI

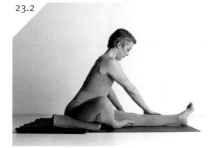

HEAD-OF-THE-KNEE POSE WITH A ROLLED
BLANKET UNDER YOUR BENT KNEE
JANU SIRSASANA

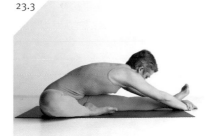

HEAD-OF-THE-KNEE POSE WITH YOUR FOOT
BACK ~ JANU SIRSASANA

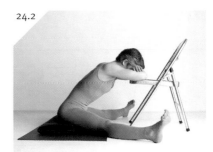

SEATED-ANGLE POSE WITH A CHAIR
UPAVISTHA KONASANA

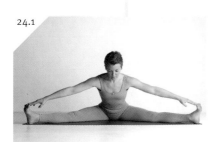

SEATED-ANGLE POSE
UPAVISTHA KONASANA

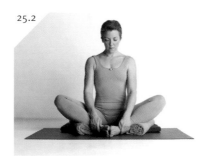

BOUND-ANGLE POSE WITH ROLLED
BLANKETS UNDER YOUR KNEES
BADDHA KONASANA

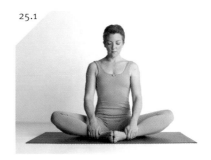

BOUND-ANGLE POSE
BADDHA KONASANA

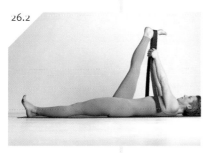

RECLINING LEG-STRETCH POSE WITH
A STRAP ~ SUPTA PADANGUSTHASANA

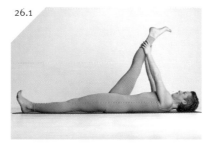

RECLINING LEG-STRETCH POSE
SUPTA PADANGUSTHASANA

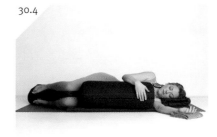

SIDE-LYING RELAXATION POSE
SAVASANA

Day Five

PURPOSE: To experience a well-rounded practice.

A WORD TO TEACHERS: Simple poses are the most satisfying to practice and to teach.

MANTRA FOR DAILY PRACTICE: Consistency is the highest form of discipline.

1.2

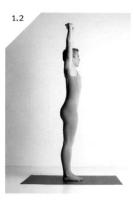

MOUNTAIN POSE
WITH YOUR ARMS OVERHEAD
TADASANA

3.3

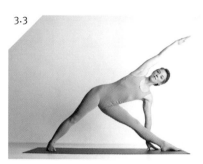

EXTENDED TRIANGLE POSE WITH YOUR ARM
OVERHEAD ~ UTTHITA TRIKONASANA

10.3

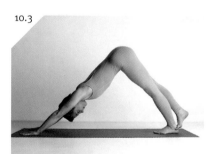

DOWNWARD-FACING DOG POSE WITH THE
TOES OF ONE FOOT ON THE HEEL OF THE
OTHER ~ ADHO MUKHA SVANASANA

3.3

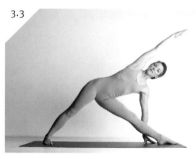

EXTENDED TRIANGLE POSE WITH YOUR ARM
OVERHEAD ~ UTTHITA TRIKONASANA

6.1

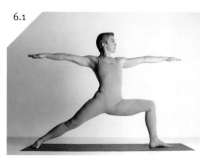

WARRIOR II POSE
VIRABHADRASANA II

7.2

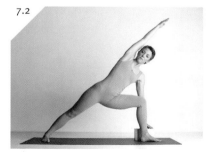

EXTENDED SIDE-ANGLE STRETCH POSE WITH
YOUR HAND ON A BLOCK
UTTHITA PARSVAKONASANA

7.3

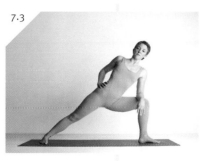

EXTENDED SIDE-ANGLE STRETCH POSE WITH
YOUR ARM SUPPORTED ON YOUR THIGH
UTTHITA PARSVAKONASANA

12.1

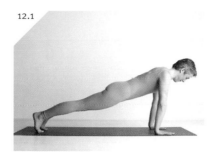

UP-PLANK POSE
CHATURANGA DANDASANA

12.3

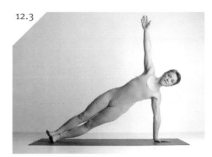

UP-PLANK POSE WITH ONE HAND UP
CHATURANGA DANDASANA

13.4

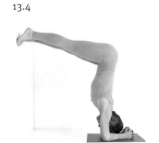

HEADSTAND PREPARATION
POSE WITH YOUR FEET ON THE
WALL ~ SALAMBA SIRSASANA

15.1

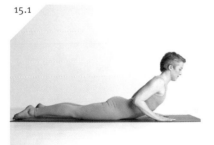

COBRA POSE
BHUJANGASANA

15.4

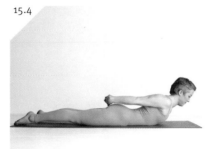

COBRA POSE WITH YOUR HANDS CLASPED
BEHIND YOUR BACK ~ BHUJANGASANA

16.3

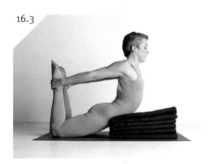

BOW POSE WITH YOUR HIPS ON BLANKETS
DHANURASANA

21.1

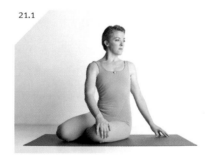

SIMPLE SEATED-TWIST POSE
BHARADVAJASANA

20.1

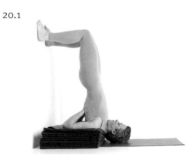

SUPPORTED SHOULDERSTAND POSE
SALAMBA SARVANGASANA

30.1

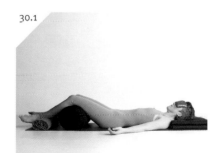

BASIC RELAXATION POSE ~ SAVASANA
WITH BREATHING PRACTICE #1: EVEN INHALATION,
EVEN EXHALATION ~ SAMA VRTTI

Day Six

PURPOSE: Opening the belly in order to open to life.

A WORD TO TEACHERS: Some studies show backbends can help prevent and even reverse osteoporosis of the vertebral column.

MANTRA FOR DAILY PRACTICE: The harder a thing is, the more it requires my softness.

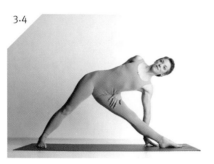

3.4

EXTENDED TRIANGLE POSE WITH YOUR ARM
BEHIND YOUR WAIST
UTTHITA TRIKONASANA

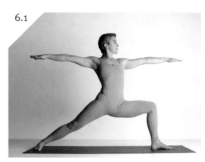

6.1

WARRIOR II POSE
VIRABHADRASANA II

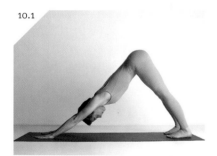

10.1

DOWNWARD-FACING DOG POSE
ADHO MUKHA SVANASANA

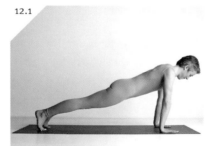

12.1

UP-PLANK POSE
CHATURANGA DANDASANA

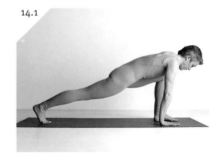

14.1

LUNGE POSE
ANJANEYASANA

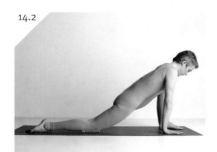

14.2

LUNGE POSE WITH YOUR BACK KNEE DOWN
ANJANEYASANA

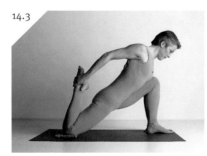

14.3

LUNGE POSE, HOLDING YOUR ANKLE
ANJANEYASANA

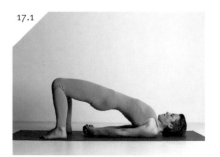

17.1

BRIDGE POSE
SETU BANDHASANA

17.2

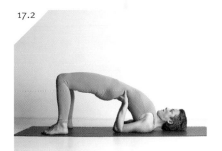

BRIDGE POSE WITH YOUR HANDS ON YOUR
BACK, FINGERS IN ~ SETU BANDHASANA

17.3

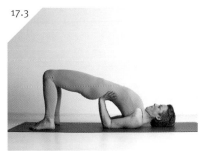

BRIDGE POSE WITH YOUR HANDS ON YOUR
BACK, FINGERS OUT ~ SETU BANDHASANA

18.1

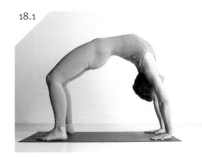

UPWARD-FACING BOW POSE
URDHVA DHANURASANA

18.2

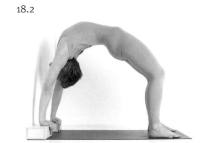

UPWARD-FACING BOW POSE AT THE WALL
AND WITH YOUR HANDS ELEVATED ON
BLOCKS ~ URDHVA DHANURASANA

18.3

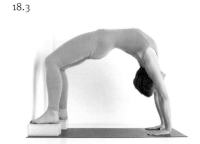

UPWARD-FACING BOW POSE AT THE WALL
AND WITH YOUR FEET ELEVATED ON BLOCKS
URDHVA DHANURASANA

17.4

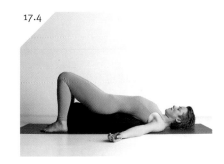

SUPPORTED BRIDGE POSE
SETU BANDHASANA

20.1

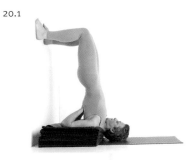

SUPPORTED SHOULDERSTAND POSE
SALAMBA SARVANGASANA

26.2

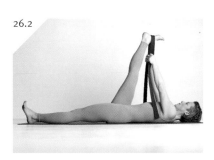

RECLINING LEG-STRETCH POSE WITH A
STRAP ~ SUPTA PADANGUSTHASANA

27.1

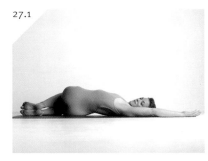

LYING TWIST POSE
JATARA PARIVARTANASANA

27.2

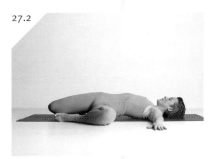

LYING TWIST POSE WITH YOUR FEET WIDE
APART ~ JATARA PARIVARTANASANA

30.3

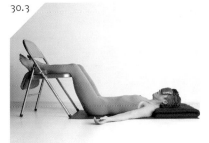

BASIC RELAXATION POSE WITH YOUR LEGS ON A CHAIR
SAVASANA ~ WITH BREATHING PRACTICE #3: SHORT
INHALATION, LONG EXHALATION ~ VISAMA VRTTI II

Day Seven

PURPOSE: To remind us to look inside for our happiness and health.

A WORD TO TEACHERS: These poses create a cool brain, which balances constant activity.

MANTRA FOR DAILY PRACTICE: Letting go is not the same thing as giving up.

10.1

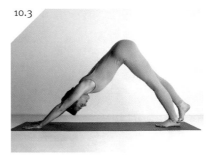

DOWNWARD–FACING DOG POSE
ADHO MUKHA SVANASANA

10.3

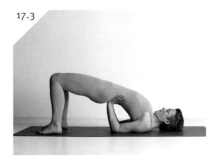

DOWNWARD-FACING DOG POSE WITH
THE TOES OF ONE FOOT ON THE HEEL OF
THE OTHER ~ ADHO MUKHA SVANASANA

9.1

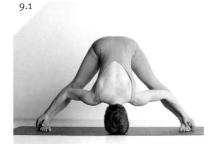

WIDE-LEG STANDING FORWARD BEND POSE
PRASARITA PADOTTANASANA

9.3

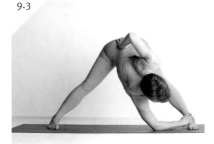

WIDE-LEG STANDING FORWARD BEND POSE
WITH A SIDE TWIST
PRASARITA PADOTTANASANA

17.3

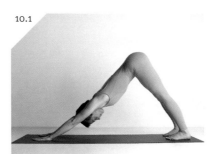

BRIDGE POSE WITH YOUR HANDS ON YOUR
BACK, FINGERS OUT ~ SETU BANDHASANA

19.1

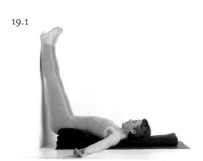

ELEVATED LEGS-UP-THE-WALL POSE
VIPARITA KARANI

24.3

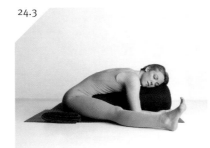

SUPPORTED SEATED-ANGLE POSE
UPAVISTHA KONASANA

25.3

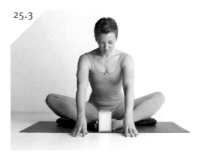

BOUND-ANGLE WITH A BLOCK BETWEEN
YOUR FEET ~ BADDHA KONASANA

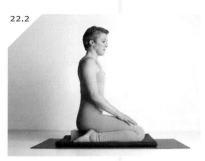

HERO–HEROINE POSE, SITTING ON A BLOCK
VIRASANA

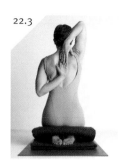

HERO–HEROINE POSE WITH
ARM STRETCH ~ VIRASANA

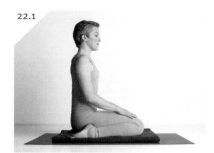

HERO–HEROINE POSE
VIRASANA

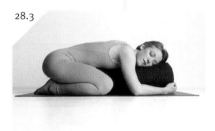

CHILD'S POSE WITH SUPPORT
ADHO MUKHA VIRASANA

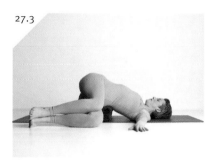

LYING TWIST POSE ON A STACK OF BLANKETS
JATARA PARIVARTANASANA

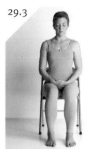

BASIC MEDITATION POSE,
SITTING ON A CHAIR
SIDDHASANA

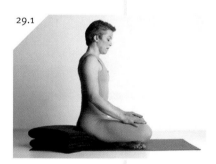

BASIC MEDITATION POSE
SIDDHASANA

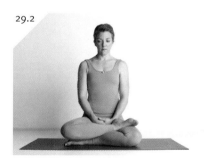

HALF-LOTUS POSE ~ ARDHA PADMASANA
(IF YOU HAVE KNEE PROBLEMS, THEN
PRACTICE FIGURE 29.4.)

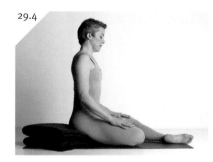

BASIC MEDITATION POSE WITH ONE LEG
ALMOST STRAIGHT ~ SIDDHASANA
(ALTERNATIVE TO FIGURE 29.2)

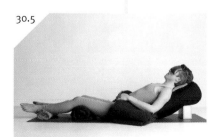

RECLINING SUPPORTED RELAXATION POSE ~ SAVASANA
WITH BREATHING PRACTICE #1: EVEN INHALATION,
EVEN EXHALATION ~ SAMA VRITI

PRACTICING WITH A SPECIFIC THEME IN MIND IS A WAY TO FOCUS ON ONE ASPECT OF YOUR BODY OR HEALTH. THE PRACTICES INCLUDED ARE FOR LOWER BACK PAIN, FOR HIP AND HAMSTRING FLEXIBILITY, FOR SHOULDER AND UPPER BACK FLEXIBILITY, FOR BALANCE, FOR STRENGTH, FOR ENERGY, FOR FATIGUE, AND FOR RELAXATION.

TEACHERS, YOU MAY FIND IT USEFUL TO TEACH ONE THEME EACH WEEK IN AN EIGHT-WEEK SERIES OF CLASSES.

Practice for Lower Back Pain

Theme Practice

PURPOSE: To relieve tension in the lower back.

A WORD TO TEACHERS: The key to a healthy back is creating and maintaining the normal curves of the spine as much as possible in all activities.

MANTRA FOR DAILY PRACTICE: I am not in charge of the universe today.

1.1

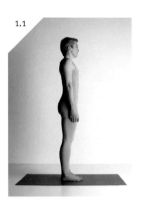

MOUNTAIN POSE
TADASANA

10.2

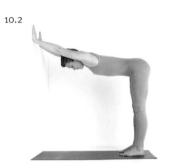

HALF-DOG POSE AT THE WALL
ADHO MUKHA SVANASANA

10.1

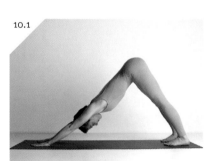

DOWNWARD-FACING DOG POSE
ADHO MUKHA SVANASANA

28.1

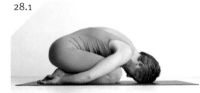

CHILD'S POSE
ADHO MUKHA VIRASANA

28.3

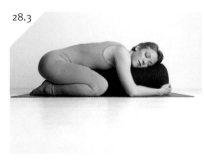

CHILD'S POSE WITH SUPPORT
ADHO MUKHA VIRASANA

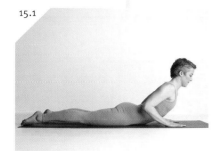

15.1

COBRA POSE
BHUJANGASANA

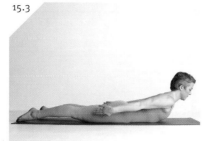

15.3

COBRA POSE WITH YOUR ARMS STRETCHED
BACKWARD ~ BHUJANGASANA

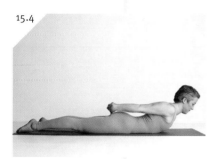

15.4

COBRA POSE WITH YOUR HANDS CLASPED
BEHIND YOUR BACK ~ BHUJANGASANA

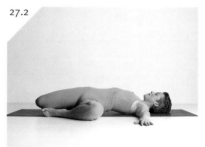

27.2

LYING TWIST POSE WITH YOUR FEET WIDE
APART ~ JATARA PARIVARTANASANA

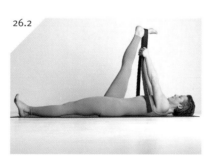

26.2

RECLINING LEG-STRETCH POSE WITH A
STRAP ~ SUPTA PADANGUSTHASANA

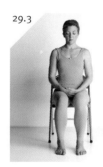

29.3

BASIC MEDITATION POSE, SITTING
ON A CHAIR ~ SIDDHASANA

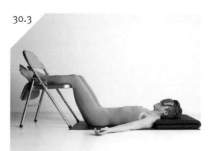

30.3

BASIC RELAXATION POSE WITH YOUR LEGS
ON A CHAIR ~ SAVASANA

Practice for Hip and Hamstring Flexibility

PURPOSE: To free up the hips for walking, running, and dancing.

A WORD TO TEACHERS: Hamstrings stretch slowly.

MANTRA FOR DAILY PRACTICE: Flexibility is a talent; adaptability is a life skill.

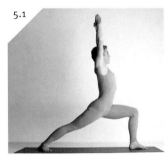

3.2

EXTENDED TRIANGLE POSE WITH YOUR HAND ON A BLOCK ~ UTTHITA TRIKONASANA

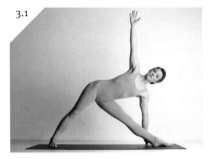

3.1

EXTENDED TRIANGLE POSE UTTHITA TRIKONASANA

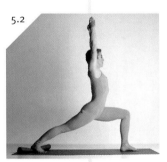

5.2

WARRIOR I POSE WITH A ROLLED MAT UNDER YOUR BACK FOOT VIRABHADRASANA I

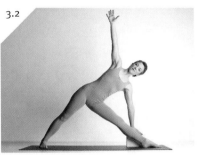

5.1

WARRIOR I POSE VIRABHADRASANA I

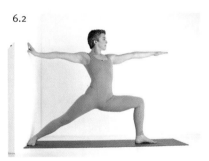

6.2

WARRIOR II POSE WITH YOUR BACK FOOT AGAINST THE WALL ~ VIRABHADRASANA II

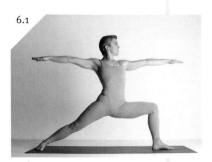

6.1

WARRIOR II POSE VIRABHADRASANA II

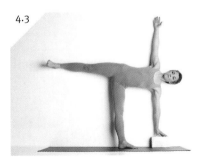

4.3

HALF-MOON POSE AT THE WALL AND WITH A BLOCK ~ ARDHA CHANDRASANA

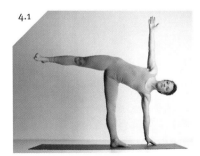

4.1

HALF-MOON POSE ARDHA CHANDRASANA

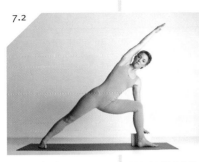

7.2

EXTENDED SIDE-ANGLE STRETCH POSE WITH
YOUR HAND ON A BLOCK
UTTHITA PARSVAKONASANA

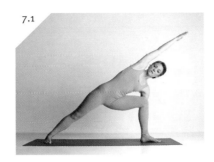

7.1

EXTENDED SIDE-ANGLE STRETCH POSE
UTTHITA PARSVAKONASANA

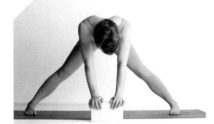

9.2

WIDE-LEG STANDING FORWARD BEND POSE
WITH A BLOCK
PRASARITA PADOTTANASANA

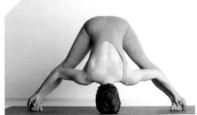

9.1

WIDE-LEG STANDING FORWARD BEND POSE
PRASARITA PADOTTANASANA

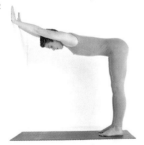

10.2

HALF-DOG POSE AT THE WALL
ADHO MUKHA SVANASANA

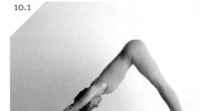

10.1

DOWNWARD-FACING DOG POSE
ADHO MUKHA SVANASANA

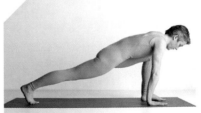

14.1

LUNGE POSE
ANJANEYASANA

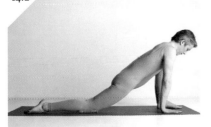

14.2

LUNGE POSE WITH YOUR BACK KNEE DOWN
ANJANEYASANA

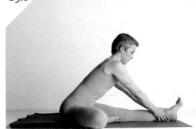

23.1

HEAD-OF-THE-KNEE POSE
JANU SIRSASANA

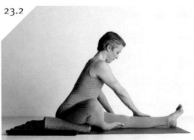

23.2

HEAD-OF-THE-KNEE POSE WITH A ROLLED
BLANKET UNDER YOUR BENT KNEE
JANU SIRSASANA

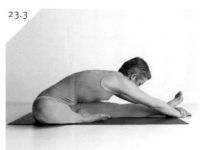

HEAD-OF-THE-KNEE POSE WITH YOUR FOOT
BACK ~ JANU SIRSASANA

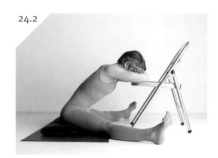

SEATED-ANGLE POSE WITH A CHAIR
UPAVISTHA KONASANA

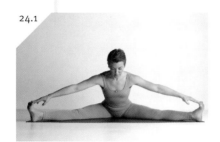

SEATED-ANGLE POSE
UPAVISTHA KONASANA

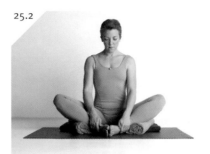

BOUND-ANGLE POSE WITH ROLLED
BLANKETS UNDER YOUR KNEES
BADDHA KONASANA

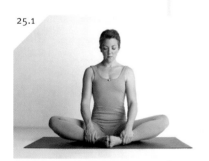

BOUND-ANGLE POSE
BADDHA KONASANA

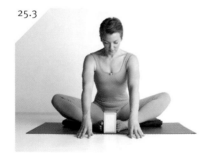

BOUND-ANGLE POSE WITH A BLOCK
BETWEEN YOUR FEET ~ BADDHA KONASANA

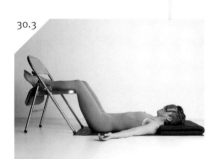

BASIC RELAXATION POSE WITH YOUR LEGS
ON A CHAIR ~ SAVASANA

Practice for Shoulder and Upper Back Flexibility

PURPOSE: To increase coordinated and free movement between the shoulder joint and the upper back.

A WORD TO TEACHERS: The strength and mobility of the upper back and shoulders influence how a person feels about her ability to affect her world through choice and action.

MANTRA FOR DAILY PRACTICE: Compassion arises in me when I feel connected with myself and with the Universe.

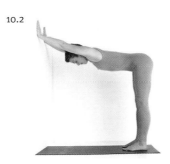

10.2

HALF-DOG POSE AT THE WALL
ADHO MUKHA SVANASANA

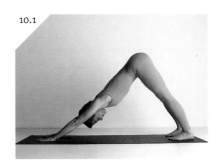

10.1

DOWNWARD-FACING DOG POSE
ADHO MUKHA SVANASANA

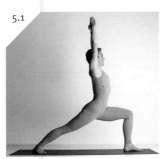

5.1

WARRIOR I POSE
VIRABHADRASANA I

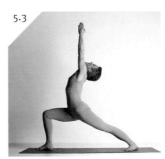

5.3

WARRIOR I POSE WITH YOUR HEAD
BACK ~ VIRABHADRASANA I

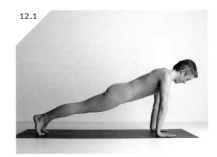

12.1

UP-PLANK POSE
CHATURANGA DANDASANA

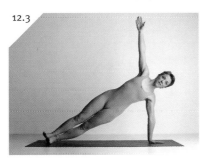

12.3

UP-PLANK POSE WITH ONE HAND UP
CHATURANGA DANDASANA

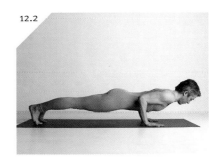

12.2

DOWN-PLANK POSE
CHATURANGA DANDASANA

13.1

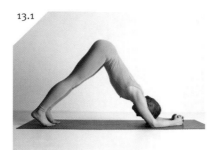

HEADSTAND PREPARATION POSE
SALAMBA SIRSASANA

13.2

13.3

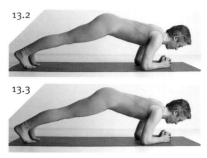

HEADSTAND PREPARATION POSE,
MOVING BACKWARD AND FORWARD
SALAMBA SIRSASANA

13.4

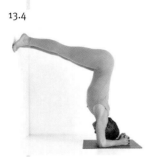

HEADSTAND PREPARATION
POSE WITH YOUR FEET ON THE
WALL ~ SALAMBA SIRSASANA

22.3

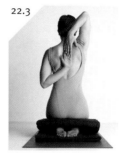

HERO–HEROINE POSE
WITH ARM STRETCH
VIRASANA

16.1

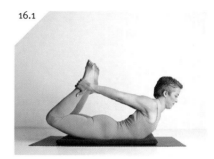

BOW POSE
DHANURASANA

16.2

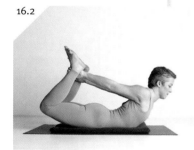

BOW POSE WITH YOUR HANDS TURNED
OUTWARD ~ DHANURASANA

16.3

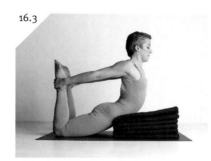

BOW POSE WITH YOUR HIPS ON BLANKETS
DHANURASANA

17.1

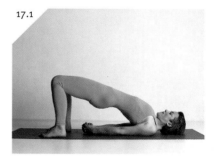

BRIDGE POSE
SETU BANDHASANA

17.4

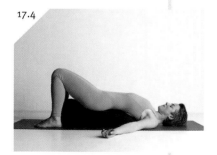

SUPPORTED BRIDGE POSE
SETU BANDHASANA

17.2

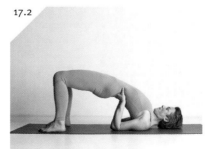

BRIDGE POSE WITH YOUR HANDS ON YOUR
BACK, FINGERS IN ~ SETU BANDHASANA

18.2

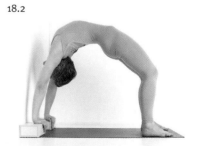

UPWARD-FACING BOW POSE AT THE WALL
AND WITH YOUR HANDS ELEVATED ON
BLOCKS ~ URDHVA DHANURASANA

18.3

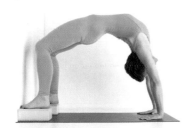

UPWARD-FACING BOW POSE AT THE WALL
AND WITH YOUR FEET ELEVATED ON BLOCKS
URDHVA DHANURASANA

18.1

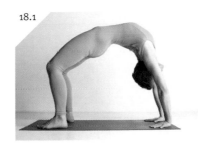

UPWARD-FACING BOW POSE
URDHVA DHANURASANA

20.1

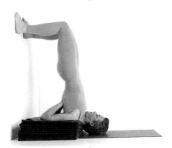

SUPPORTED SHOULDERSTAND POSE
SALAMBA SARVANGASANA

20.2

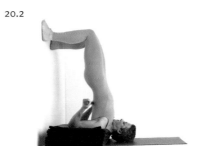

SUPPORTED SHOULDERSTAND POSE WITH A
POLE ~ SALAMBA SARVANGASANA

27.1

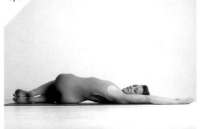

LYING TWIST POSE
JATARA PARIVARTANASANA

27.2

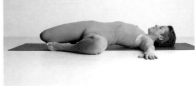

LYING TWIST POSE WITH YOUR FEET WIDE
APART ~ JATARA PARIVARTANASANA

27.3

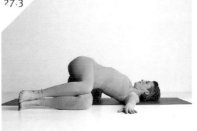

LYING TWIST POSE ON A STACK OF
BLANKETS ~ JATARA PARIVARTANASANA

30.2

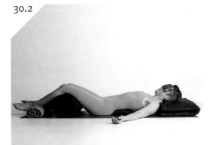

BASIC RELAXATION POSE WITH BACK
SUPPORT ~ SAVASANA

Practice for Balance

PURPOSE: To improve balance in the new student and to prevent its loss in the experienced one.

A WORD TO TEACHERS: Balance is the key to a life well lived.

MANTRA FOR DAILY PRACTICE: The opposite of instability is not certainty: it is faith.

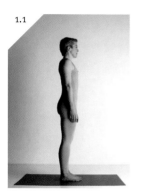

MOUNTAIN POSE
TADASANA

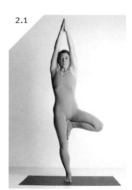

TREE POSE
VRKSASANA

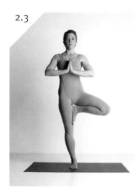

TREE POSE WITH YOUR HANDS
IN NAMASTE ~ VRKSASANA

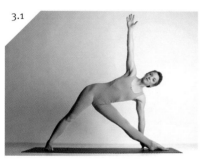

EXTENDED TRIANGLE POSE
UTTHITA TRIKONASANA

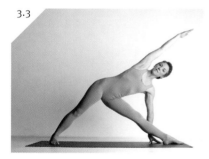

EXTENDED TRIANGLE POSE WITH YOUR ARM
OVERHEAD ~ UTTHITA TRIKONASANA

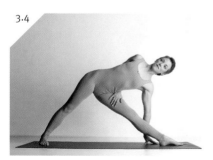

EXTENDED TRIANGLE POSE WITH YOUR ARM
BEHIND YOUR WAIST
UTTHITA TRIKONASANA

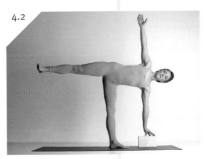

4.2

HALF-MOON POSE WITH YOUR HAND ON
A BLOCK ~ ARDHA CHANDRASANA

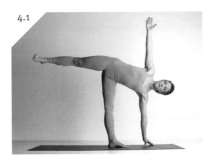

4.1

HALF-MOON POSE
ARDHA CHANDRASANA

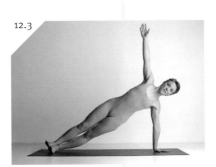

5.3

WARRIOR I POSE WITH YOUR
HEAD BACK ~ VIRABHADRASANA I

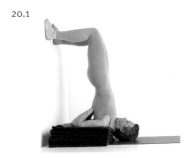

12.1

UP-PLANK POSE
CHATURANGA DANDASANA

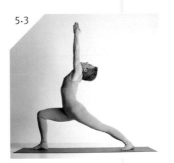

12.3

UP-PLANK POSE WITH ONE HAND UP
CHATURANGA DANDASANA

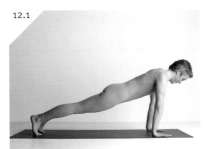

13.4

HEADSTAND PREPARATION POSE
WITH YOUR FEET ON THE WALL
SALAMBA SIRSASANA

20.1

SUPPORTED SHOULDERSTAND POSE
SALAMBA SARVANGASANA

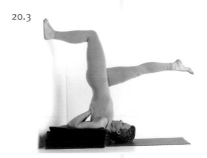

20.3

ONE-LEGGED SHOULDERSTAND POSE
SALAMBA SARVANGASANA

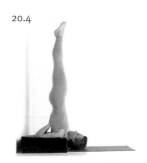

20.4

BALANCING IN SUPPORTED
SHOULDERSTAND POSE
SALAMBA SARVANGASANA

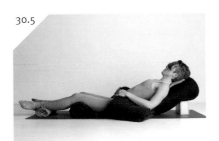

30.5

RECLINING SUPPORTED RELAXATION POSE
SAVASANA

Practice for Strength

PURPOSE: To understand that strength can be manifested in more than physical ways.

A WORD TO TEACHERS: Strong arms create confidence and courage.

MANTRA FOR DAILY PRACTICE: One good laugh is worth a thousand right answers.

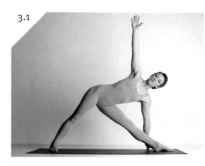

3.1

EXTENDED TRIANGLE POSE
UTTHITA TRIKONASANA

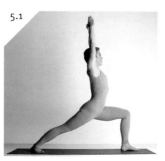

5.1

WARRIOR I POSE
VIRABHADRASANA I

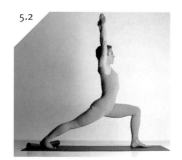

5.2

WARRIOR I POSE WITH A ROLLED
MAT UNDER YOUR BACK FOOT
VIRABHADRASANA I

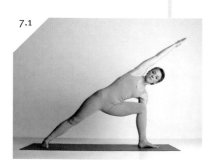

7.1

EXTENDED SIDE-ANGLE STRETCH POSE
UTTHITA PARSVAKONASANA

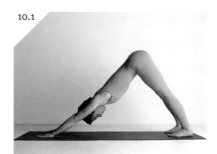

10.1

DOWNWARD-FACING DOG POSE
ADHO MUKHA SVANASANA

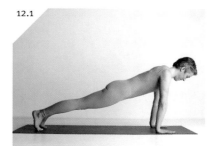

12.1

UP-PLANK POSE
CHATURANGA DANDASANA

12.2

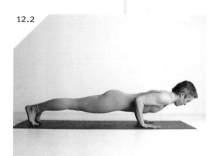

DOWN-PLANK POSE
CHATURANGA DANDASANA

13.1

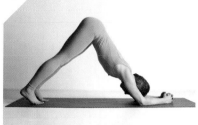

HEADSTAND PREPARATION POSE
SALAMBA SIRSASANA

13.2

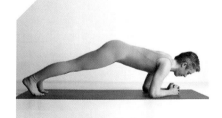

13.3

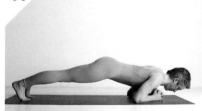

HEADSTAND PREPARATION POSE, MOVING BACKWARD AND FORWARD
SALAMBA SIRSASANA

13.4

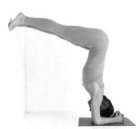

HEADSTAND PREPARATION
POSE WITH YOUR FEET ON THE
WALL ~ SALAMBA SIRSASANA

30.1

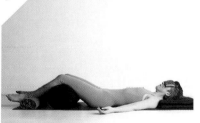

BASIC RELAXATION POSE
SAVASANA

Practice for Energy

PURPOSE: To free up your own natural energy.

A WORD TO TEACHERS: Energy is always available to a person when he remembers his deep connection to the whole.

MANTRA FOR DAILY PRACTICE: Practice allows me to gain access to the energy that is already inside me.

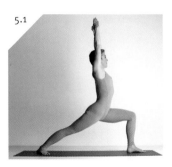

5.1

WARRIOR I POSE
VIRABHADRASANA I

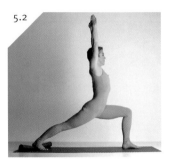

5.2

WARRIOR I POSE WITH A
ROLLED MAT UNDER YOUR BACK
FOOT ~ VIRABHADRASANA I

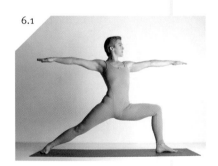

6.1

WARRIOR II POSE
VIRABHADRASANA II

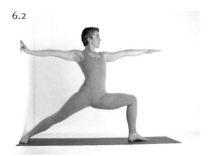

6.2

WARRIOR II POSE WITH YOUR BACK FOOT
AGAINST THE WALL ~ VIRABHADRASANA II

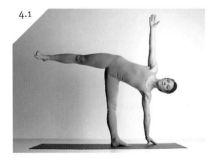

4.1

HALF-MOON POSE
ARDHA CHANDRASANA

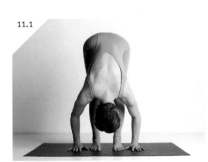

11.1

STANDING FORWARD BEND POSE
UTTANASANA

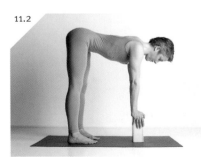

11.2

STANDING FORWARD BEND POSE WITH
YOUR HANDS ON A BLOCK ~ UTTANASANA

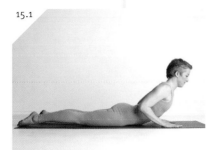

15.1

COBRA POSE
BHUJANGASANA

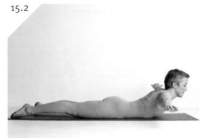

15.2

COBRA POSE WITH YOUR ARMS STRETCHED
TO THE SIDES ~ BHUJANGASANA

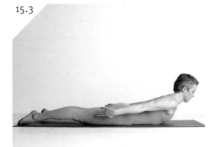

15.3

COBRA POSE WITH YOUR ARMS STRETCHED
BACKWARD ~ BHUJANGASANA

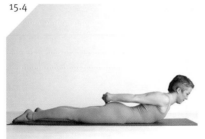

15.4

COBRA POSE WITH YOUR HANDS CLASPED
BEHIND YOUR BACK ~ BHUJANGASANA

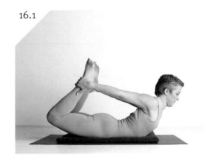

16.1

BOW POSE
DHANURASANA

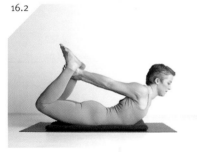

16.2

BOW POSE WITH YOUR HANDS TURNED OUT-
WARD ~ DHANURASANA

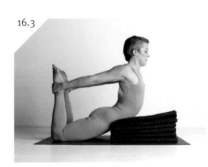

16.3

BOW POSE WITH YOUR HIPS ON BLANKETS
DHANURASANA

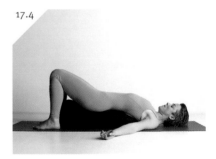

17.4

SUPPORTED BRIDGE POSE
SETU BANDHASANA

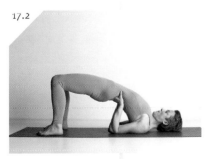

17.2

BRIDGE POSE WITH YOUR HANDS ON YOUR
BACK, FINGERS IN ~ SETU BANDHASANA

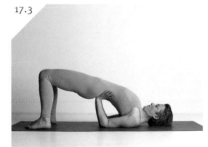

17.3

BRIDGE POSE WITH YOUR HANDS ON YOUR
BACK, FINGERS OUT ~ SETU BANDHASANA

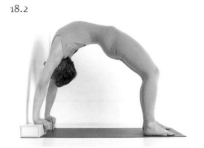

18.2

UPWARD-FACING BOW POSE AT THE WALL
AND WITH YOUR HANDS ELEVATED ON
BLOCKS ~ URDHVA DHANURASANA

228

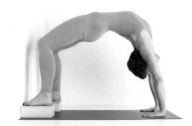

18.3

UPWARD-FACING BOW POSE AT THE WALL
AND WITH YOUR FEET ELEVATED ON BLOCKS
URDHVA DHANURASANA

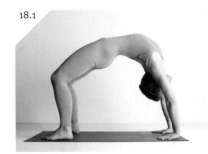

18.1

UPWARD-FACING BOW POSE
URDHVA DHANURASANA

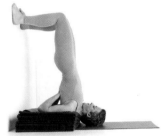

20.1

SUPPORTED SHOULDERSTAND POSE
SALAMBA SARVANGASANA

20.2

SUPPORTED SHOULDERSTAND POSE WITH A
POLE ~ SALAMBA SARVANGASANA

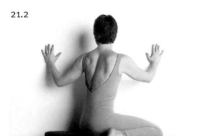

21.2

SIMPLE SEATED-TWIST POSE AT THE WALL
BHARADVAJASANA

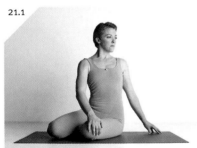

21.1

SIMPLE SEATED-TWIST POSE
BHARADVAJASANA

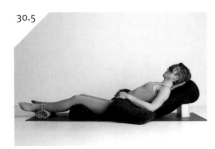

30.5

RECLINING SUPPORTED RELAXATION POSE ~ SAVASANA
WITH BREATHING PRACTICE #2: LONG INHALATION,
SHORT EXHALATION ~ VISAMA VRTTI I

Practice for Fatigue

PURPOSE: To learn the importance of doing less.

A WORD TO TEACHERS: It is not what a person does, but who she is, that enriches her life.

MANTRA FOR DAILY PRACTICE: Everyone who is alive has exactly the same amount of time today.

9.2

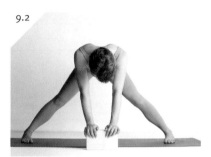

WIDE-LEG STANDING FORWARD BEND POSE
WITH A BLOCK
PRASARITA PADOTTANASANA

9.1

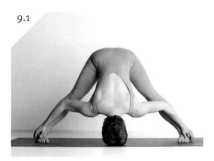

WIDE-LEG STANDING FORWARD BEND POSE
PRASARITA PADOTTANASANA

9.3

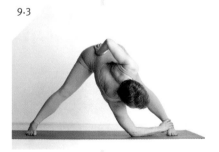

WIDE-LEG STANDING FORWARD BEND POSE
WITH A SIDE TWIST
PRASARITA PADOTTANASANA

10.2

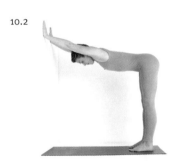

HALF-DOG POSE AT THE WALL
ADHO MUKHA SVANASANA

19.1

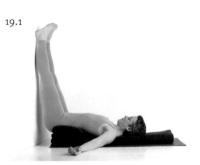

ELEVATED LEGS-UP-THE-WALL POSE
VIPARITA KARANI

19.2

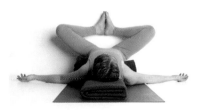

ELEVATED LEGS-UP-THE-WALL POSE WITH
LEGS IN BOUND-ANGLE POSE
VIPARITA KARANI

19.3

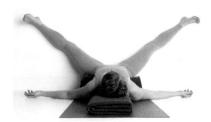

ELEVATED LEGS-UP-THE-WALL POSE WITH
LEGS IN SEATED-ANGLE POSE
VIPARITA KARANI

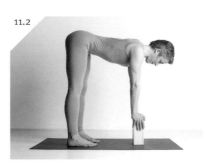

STANDING FORWARD BEND POSE WITH YOUR
HANDS ON A BLOCK ~ UTTANASANA

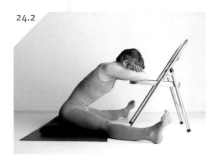

HERO–HEROINE POSE, SITTING ON A BLOCK
VIRASANA

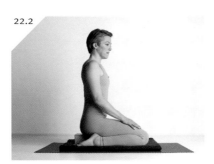

HERO–HEROINE POSE
VIRASANA

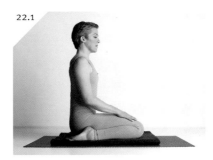

SEATED-ANGLE POSE WITH A CHAIR
UPAVISTHA KONASANA

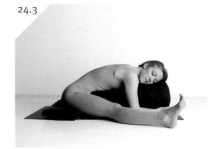

SUPPORTED SEATED-ANGLE POSE
UPAVISTHA KONASANA

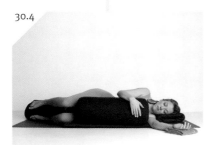

SIDE-LYING RELAXATION POSE
SAVASANA

Practice for Relaxation

PURPOSE: To learn the healthy joy of doing less.

A WORD TO TEACHERS: Resting is as important as stretching.

MANTRA FOR DAILY PRACTICE: Just for today, I will do everything 10 percent slower.

11.1

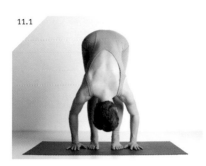

STANDING FORWARD BEND POSE
UTTANASANA

11.2

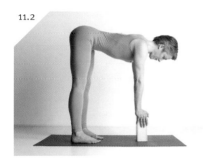

STANDING FORWARD BEND POSE WITH YOUR
HANDS ON A BLOCK ~ UTTANASANA

19.1

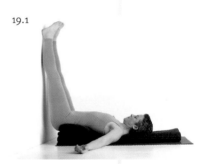

ELEVATED LEGS-UP-THE-WALL POSE
VIPARITA KARANI

19.2

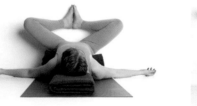

ELEVATED LEGS-UP-THE-WALL POSE WITH
LEGS IN BOUND-ANGLE POSE
VIPARITA KARANI

19.3

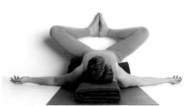

ELEVATED LEGS-UP-THE-WALL POSE WITH
LEGS IN SEATED-ANGLE POSE
VIPARITA KARANI

23.1

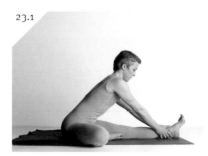

HEAD-OF-THE-KNEE POSE
JANU SIRSASANA

23.2

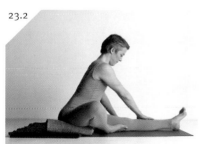

HEAD-OF-THE-KNEE POSE WITH A ROLLED
BLANKET UNDER YOUR BENT KNEE
JANU SIRSASANA

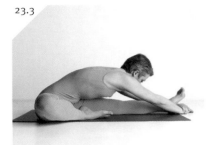

HEAD-OF-THE-KNEE POSE WITH YOUR FOOT
BACK ~ JANU SIRSASANA

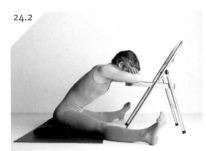

SEATED-ANGLE POSE WITH A CHAIR
UPAVISTHA KONASANA

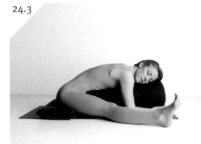

SUPPORTED SEATED-ANGLE POSE
UPAVISTHA KONASANA

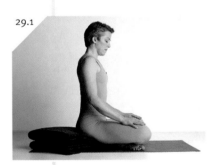

BASIC MEDITATION POSE
SIDDHASANA

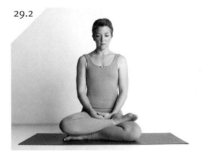

HALF-LOTUS POSE
ARDHA PADMASANA

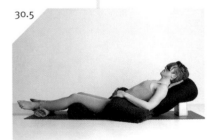

RECLINING SUPPORTED RELAXATION POSE
SAVASANA ~ WITH BREATHING PRACTICE #1:
EVEN INHALATION, EVEN EXHALATION ~ SAMA VRTTI

The 30 Essential Yoga Poses Practice

PURPOSE: To integrate all the basic poses into one practice.

A WORD TO TEACHERS: Understanding and sharing these poses is the heart of yoga teaching.

MANTRA FOR DAILY PRACTICE: The way I *do* my yoga practice is the way that I *do* my life.

1.1

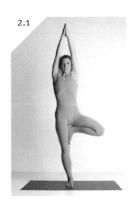

MOUNTAIN POSE
TADASANA

2.1

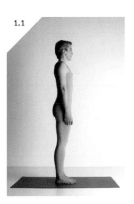

TREE POSE
VRKSASANA

3.1

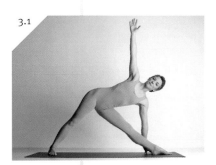

EXTENDED TRIANGLE POSE
UTTHITA TRIKONASANA

4.1

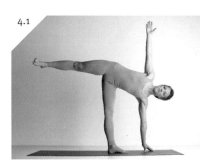

HALF-MOON POSE
ARDHA CHANDRASANA

5.1

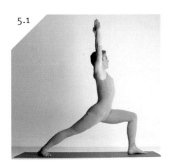

WARRIOR I POSE
VIRABHADRASANA I

6.1

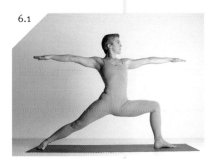

WARRIOR II POSE
VIRABHADRASANA II

7.1

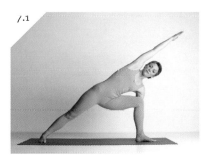

EXTENDED SIDE-ANGLE STRETCH POSE
UTTHITA PARSVAKONASANA

8.1

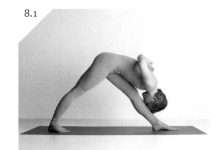

SIDE-CHEST STRETCH POSE
PARSVOTTANASANA

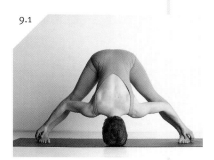

WIDE-LEG STANDING FORWARD BEND POSE
PRASARITA PADOTTANASANA

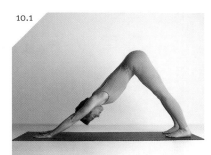

DOWNWARD-FACING DOG POSE
ADHO MUKHA SVANASANA

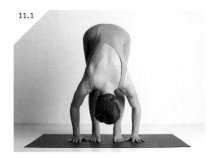

STANDING FORWARD BEND POSE
UTTANASANA

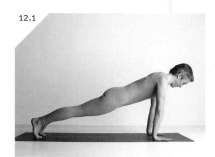

UP-PLANK POSE
CHATURANAGA DANDASANA

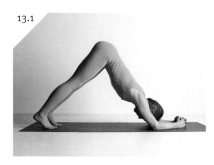

HEADSTAND PREPARATION POSE
SALAMBA SIRSASANA

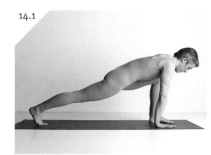

LUNGE POSE
ANJANEYASANA

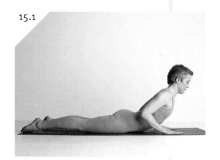

COBRA POSE
BHUJANGASANA

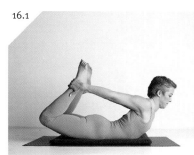

BOW POSE
DHANURASANA

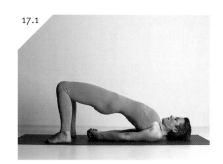

BRIDGE POSE
SETU BANDHASANA

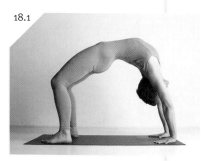

UPWARD-FACING BOW POSE
URDHVA DHANURASANA

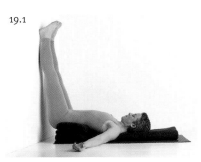

ELEVATED LEGS-UP-THE-WALL POSE
VIPARITA KARANI

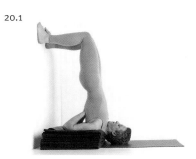

SUPPORTED SHOULDERSTAND POSE
SALAMBA SARVANGASANA

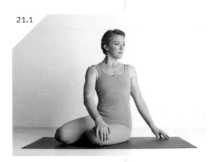

SIMPLE SEATED-TWIST POSE
BHARADVAJASANA

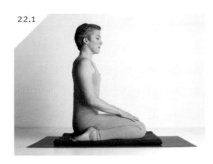

HERO–HEROINE POSE
VIRASANA

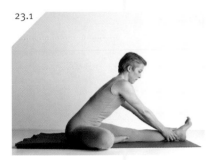

HEAD-OF-THE-KNEE POSE
JANU SIRSASANA

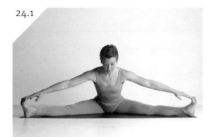

SEATED-ANGLE POSE
UPAVISTHA KONASANA

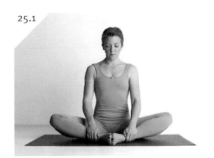

BOUND-ANGLE POSE
BADDHA KONASANA

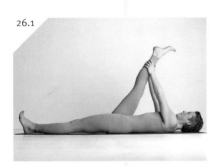

RECLINING LEG-STRETCH POSE
SUPTA PADANGUSTHASANA

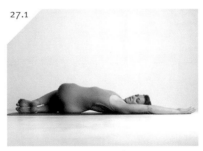

LYING TWIST POSE
JATARA PARIVARTANASANA

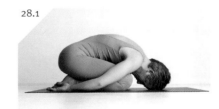

CHILD'S POSE
ADHO MUKHA VIRASANA

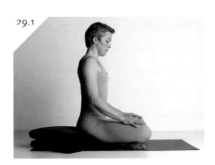

BASIC MEDITATION POSE
SIDDHASANA

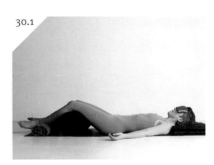

BASIC RELAXATION POSE
SAVASANA

PART FIVE

AND MORE

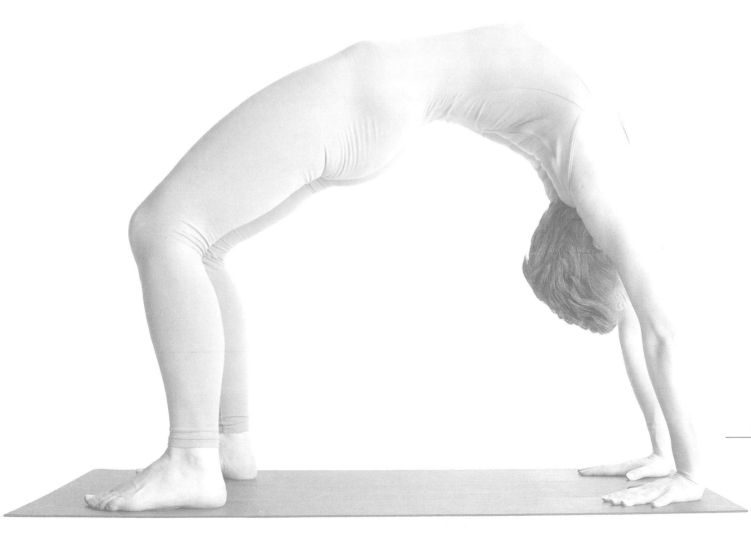

237

Glossary

Achilles tendon. The large tendon of the calf muscle, located at the back of the ankle. It attaches the calf muscle to the heel bone.

Adduct or adduction. To move toward the midline of the body.

Adductors or adductor muscles. The muscles of the inner thigh. When they contract, they bring the thighs together.

Calf muscles. The muscles of the back of the lower leg.

Cervical spine. The seven bones of the neck.

Coccyx. Tailbone.

Concave. Rounded inward.

Convex. Rounded outward.

Detached retina. The separation of the inner sensory layer of the retina from the outer layer that leads to a loss of retinal function.

Diaphragm. The driving muscle of respiration that divides the thorax and the abdomen.

Disc disease. The degeneration of the discs between the vertebrae of the spine.

Erector muscles. The long muscles along the vertebral column that extend or backbend the spinal column.

Extension. The opening or straightening of a joint; the opposite of flexion.

External rotators. See "Rotators."

Femur. Thighbone.

Flexion. The closing of a joint; the opposite of extension.

Glaucoma. An increase in eye pressure that can result in a wasting of the optic nerve and blindness.

Gleno-humeral rhythm. A series of coordinated movements involving the shoulder joint, collarbone, and midback area, which allow for full flexion and full abduction of the shoulder joint.

Gluteus Maximus. The large external muscle of the buttocks that, when contracted, extends and externally rotates the femur.

Hamstrings. The long muscles of the back of the thigh that flex the knee and extend the hip. They are named the semimenbranosus, the semitendinosus, and the biceps femoris.

Hiatal hernia. The protrusion of part of the stomach through an opening in the diaphragm.

Hipbones. This term refers to the pelvic bones, usually the ilium, the largest and flattest bone of the pelvis.

Hip extension. The movement of the hip joint in which the femur is taken backward, as occurs in a backbend.

Hip flexors. The muscles of the front top thigh that create hip flexion, which is the movement of the thigh toward the trunk.

Hyperextension. The movement of joints, usually the elbow joints or the knee joints, past their normal range of extension.

Hypertension. Consistent blood pressure readings that are higher than 140/90.

Ilium. See "Hipbones."

Intercostals. The small muscles between the ribs that move during respiration.

Intrascapular muscles. The muscles between the scapulae, which draw these bones together and frequently stabilize them during large and strong movements of the arm and shoulder.

Ligament. A connective tissue that connects bone to bone.

Low blood pressure. Consistently low blood pressure readings, generally considered to be readings below 120/80.

Lumbar spine. The five vertebrae of the lower back, found between the bottom rib and the top back rim of the pelvis.

Nutation. A small, involuntary, and forward (to the front of the body) movement of the first sacral vertebra, which accompanies extension, or backbending, of the lumbar spine.

Pectorals or pectoralis muscles. The muscles of the upper, outer chest wall, which adduct the arm toward the trunk.

Pelvis. The basin-shaped structure of the lower extremity that is made up of the ilia, ischiums, pubic bones, sacrum, and coccyx. The word *basin* comes from the Latin word *bacca*, which means "water vessel."

Pubic bone. The front, lower bone of the pelvis.

Quadriceps femoris or quadriceps muscles. The large, four-headed muscles of the front thigh that both straighten the thigh and help in flexing the hip joint.

Quadriceps tendon. The tendon that crosses the patella (kneecap) and attaches the quadriceps muscles to the front of the tibia (shin).

Repetitive strain injury (RSI). Swelling of the tendons on the inside of the wrist, causing pain and usually created by overuse.

Rotators. The muscles of the lateral hip joint that externally rotate the thigh.

Sacroiliac joint. The articulation of the ilium of the pelvis with the sacrum bone of the spinal column, the main function of which is stability.

Sacrum. The outwardly curved bone at the base of the spinal column, which consists of five fused vertebrae.

Scapulae. The two shoulder blades.

Sciatica. The irritation of the sciatic nerve in the back of the thigh caused by compression on that nerve.

Spinal column. The backbone, also known as the vertebral column.

Spondylolistheses. The forward slipping of a lower lumbar vertebrae on the sacrum.

Spondylolysis. The breakdown of a vertebral structure, especially the body of the vertebrae, that usually occurs in the lower lumbar spine.

Thoracic spine. The middle of the spine, consisting of twelve vertebrae, which are attached to the ribs.

Triceps. The muscles of the back upper arm that straighten the elbow and help to extend the arm.

Trimester. A division of pregnancy.

Resources

YOGA WITH JUDITH LASATER

Judith Lasater offers ongoing yoga classes, leads yoga vacations, lectures and teaches at yoga conferences, and gives workshops and seminars, including Relax and Renew Seminars® and Living Your Yoga Seminars®. All are open to interested individuals, yoga teachers, and health care professionals. For more information, visit www.judithlasater.com.

BOOKS

Lasater, Judith, Ph.D., P.T. *Living Your Yoga: Finding the Spiritual in Everyday Life.* Berkeley, Calif.: Rodmell Press, 2000. (800) 841–3123, www.rodmellpress.com.

———. *Relax and Renew: Restful Yoga for Stressful Times.* Berkeley, Calif.: Rodmell Press, 1995. (800) 841–3123, www.rodmellpress.com.

MANTRA MATS™

Inspire your yoga practice with Judith Lasater's Mantra Mats™. Each mat is silk-screened with a "Mantra for Daily Living," from her *Living Your Yoga.* For more information, contact Hugger-Mugger Yoga Products at (800) 473–4888, www.huggermugger.com.

CHAIR, CLOTHING, AND PROPS PHOTOGRAPHED IN *30 ESSENTIAL YOGA POSES*

Chair: Meco Corporation, (800) 251–7558, www.meco.net

Clothing: Marie Wright Yoga Wear, (800) 217–0006, www.mariewright.com

Props: Hugger-Mugger Yoga Products, (800) 473–4888, www.huggermugger.com

OTHER RECOMMENDED RESOURCES

BOOKS

Feuerstein, Georg, Ph.D. *The Yoga Tradition: History, Religion, Philosophy, and Practice* (unabridged, new format edition). Prescott, Ariz.: Hohm Press, 2001.

Miller, Barbara Stoller (translator). *Yoga: Discipline of Freedom: The Yoga Sutra Attributed to Patanjali.* New York: Bantam Doubleday Dell, 1998.

Rutter, Peter, M.D. *Sex in the Forbidden Zone: When Men in Power—Therapists, Doctors, Clergy, Teachers, and Others—Betray Women's Trust.* New York: Ballantine Books, 1997.

MAGAZINES

The following yoga periodicals have published articles by Judith Lasater:

Ascent ✦ www.ascentmagazine.com

LA Yoga ✦ www.layogapages.com

Yoga Chicago ✦ www.yogachicago.com

Yoga International ✦ www.yimag.org

Yoga Journal ✦ www.yogajournal.com

SPOKEN AUDIO

Schatz, Mary Pullig, M.D. *Relaxation.* Available from Rodmell Press, (800) 841–3123, www.rodmellpress.com.

CALIFORNIA YOGA TEACHERS ASSOCIATION CODE OF ETHICS

www.yogateachersassoc.org

WHERE TO FIND A YOGA TEACHER ONLINE

www.yogaalliance.com ✦ www.yogajournal.com ✦ www.yogateachersassoc.org

About the Model

THERESA ELLIOTT began her study of yoga in 1987, after a decade of study in music and dance. In 1990, she was certified to teach yoga in the tradition of B. K. S. Iyengar. She has gone on to work extensively with asana in movement. Core work, unique movement patterns, and humor are the heart of her teaching.

In 1995, she produced the video entitled *Stillness in Motion: Yoga Vinyasa;* she was featured in the *Yoga Journal 1996 Calendar.* She serves as a spokesperson for Hugger-Mugger Yoga Products. She is an avid ballroom dancer, and greatly enjoys life with her daughter.

She teaches full time at The Yoga Tree, in Seattle, Washington, where she is also the director of the teacher training program. In addition, she gives workshops throughout the United States. For more information about Theresa Elliott's teaching and video, visit www.yogatree.com or send an e-mail to mercuryyoga@seanet.com.

About the Author

Judith Lasater has taught yoga since 1971. She holds a doctorate in East–West psychology and is a physical therapist. She is president of the California Yoga Teachers Association, and serves on the advisory boards of *Yoga Journal* and the Yoga Research and Education Center.

Her yoga training includes study with B. K. S. Iyengar in India and the United States. She teaches yoga classes and trains yoga teachers in kinesiology, yoga therapeutics, and the Yoga Sutra in the San Francisco Bay Area. She also gives workshops throughout the United States, and has taught in Canada, England, France, Indonesia, Japan, Mexico, Peru, and Russia.

She writes extensively on the therapeutic aspects of yoga. Her best-selling *Relax and Renew: Restful Yoga for Stressful Times* (Rodmell Press, 1995) is the first book devoted exclusively to the supported yoga poses and breathing techniques that make up restorative yoga. Her second book is entitled *Living Your Yoga: Finding the Spiritual in Everyday Life* (Rodmell Press, 2000).

Her popular "Asana" column ran in *Yoga Journal* for thirteen years, and she continues to contribute articles on a variety of subjects. In addition, her writing has appeared in numerous magazines and books, including *Yoga International, Natural Health, Sports Illustrated for Women, Prevention, Alternative Therapies, Numedx, International Journal of Yoga Therapy* (formerly *The Journal of the International Association of Yoga Therapists*), *Complementary Therapies in Rehabilitation* (Slack), *Living Yoga* (Jeremy P. Tarcher/Perigee), *American Yoga* (Grove Press), *The New Yoga for People Over 50* (Health Communications), *and Lilias, Yoga, and Your Life* (Macmillan).

Judith Lasater lives in the San Francisco Bay Area with her family.

Yoga with Judith Lasater, Ph.D., P.T.

Judith Lasater offers ongoing yoga classes, leads yoga vacations, lectures and teaches at yoga conferences, and gives workshops and seminars, including Relax and Renew Seminars® and Living Your Yoga Seminars®. All are open to interested individuals, yoga teachers, and health care professionals. For more information about her teaching schedule, visit www.judithlasater.com.

From the Publisher

Rodmell Press publishes books on yoga, Buddhism, and aikido. In the Bhagavadgita it is written, "Yoga is skill in action." It is our hope that our books will help individuals develop a more skillful practice— one that brings peace to their daily lives and to the Earth.

We thank all whose support, encouragement, and practical advice sustain us in our efforts. In particular, we are grateful to Reb Anderson, B. K. S. Iyengar, and Yvonne Rand for their inspiration.

CATALOG REQUEST
Rodmell Press
(510) 841–3123, (800) 841-3123
(510) 841–3191 (fax)
info@rodmellpress.com
www.rodmellpress.com

TRADE SALES
Australia
Banyan Tree Book Distributors
+61–(0)–8-8363–4244
+61–(0)–8-8363–4255 (fax)
sales@banyantreebooks.com.au
www.banyantreebooks.com.au

Canada
SCB Distributors
(310) 532–9400, (800) 729-6423
(310) 532–7001 (fax)
info@scbdistributors.com
www.scbdistributors.com

New Zealand
Addenda
+64–9-836–7471
+64–9-836–7401 (fax)
addenda@addenda.co.nz

South Africa
Titles
+27–11-880–9634
+27–11-447–5377 (fax)
vicsaunder@iafrica.com

United Kingdom/Europe
Wisdom Books
+44–(0)–208-553–5020
+44–(0)–208-553–5122 (fax)
sales@wisdom-books.com
www.wisdom-books.com

United States
SCB Distributors
(310) 532–9400, (800) 729-6423
(310) 532–7001 (fax)
info@scbdistributors.com
www.scbdistributors.com

FOREIGN LANGUAGE AND BOOK CLUB RIGHTS
Donald Moyer, Publisher
(510) 841–3123
donald@rodmellpress.com
www.rodmellpress.com

Index

Adho Mukha Svanasana. See Downward-Facing Dog Pose
Adho Mukha Virasana. See Child's Pose
Anjaneyasana. See Lunge Pose
Ardha Chandrasana. See Half-Moon Pose
Ardha Padmasana (Half-Lotus Pose), 181, 213, 232
asana. *See also specific poses*
  as limb of classical yoga, 2, 13
  sequencing, 3, 196–197
  time to hold poses, 198

back, practices for, 214–215, 219–221
Baddha Konasana. See Bound-Angle Pose
balance, 222–223
Basic Meditation Pose (*Siddhasana*)
  in back pain practice, 215
  in Day-of-Week Practice, 213
  overview, 179–183
  in relaxation practice, 232
  in 30 Poses Practice, 235
  variation: Half-Lotus, 181, 213, 232
  variation: one leg almost straight, 182, 183, 213
  variation: sitting on chair, 182, 213, 215
Basic Relaxation Pose (*Savasana*)
  allowing time for, 198
  in back pain practice, 215
  in balance practice, 223
  in Busy Days Practice, 199
  in Day-of-Week Practice, 201, 203, 205, 207, 209, 211, 213
  in energy practice, 228
  in fatigue practice, 230
  in flexibility practice, 218, 221
  overview, 185–191
  in relaxation practice, 232
  in strength practice, 225
  in 30 Poses Practice, 235
  variation: legs on chair, 188–189, 201, 205, 211, 215, 218
  variation: reclining supported, 190, 213, 223, 228, 232
  variation: side-lying, 189, 207, 230
  variation: with back support, 187–188, 203, 221

Bharadvajasana. See Simple Seated-Twist Pose
Bhujangasana. See Cobra Pose
blanket, standard fold, 187
Bolen, Jean Shinoda, 7
Bound-Angle Pose (*Baddha Konasana*)
  in Day of Week Practice, 207, 212
  in flexibility practice, 218
  overview, 157–161
  in 30 Poses Practice, 235
  variation: block between feet, 160, 161, 212, 218
  variation: rolled blanket under knees, 160, 207, 218
boundaries, 6–7, 10–11, 12
Bow Pose (*Dhanurasana*)
  in Day-of-Week Practice, 205, 209
  in energy practice, 227
  in flexibility practice, 220
  overview, 103–107
  in 30 Poses Practice, 234
  variation: hands turned outward, 105–106, 220, 227
  variation: hips on blankets, 106, 209, 220, 227
Breathing Practices. *See* Essential Breathing Practices (*Pranayama*)
Bridge Pose (*Setu Bandhasana*)
  in Day-of-Week Practice, 201, 205, 210–211, 212
  in energy practice, 227
  in flexibility practice, 220
  overview, 109–113
  in 30 Poses Practice, 234
  variation: hands on back, fingers in, 111, 211, 220, 227
  variation: hands on back, fingers out, 112, 211, 212, 227
  variation: supported, 112, 113, 211, 220, 227
Busy Days Practice, 199

California Yoga Teachers Association Code of Ethics, 241
Chaturanga Dandasana. See Up-Plank Pose and Down-Plank Pose
Child's Pose (*Adho Mukha Virasana*)

in back pain practice, 214
in Day-of-Week Practice, 203, 213
overview, 175–177
in 30 Poses Practice, 235
variation: blanket on heels, 176–177, 203
variation: with support, 177, 213, 214
classes
  ending in Namaste, 196
  guidelines for students, 8–9
  guidelines for teachers, 9–11
  from Judith Lasater, 240, 243
  sacred circle for, 7, 196
  sequencing for, 3
clothing, 8, 10, 240
Cobra Pose (*Bhujangasana*)
  in back pain practice, 215
  in Day-of-Week Practice, 204–205, 209
  in energy practice, 227
  overview, 97–101
  in 30 Poses Practice, 234
  variation: arms backward, 100, 204, 215, 227
  variation: arms to sides, 99, 204, 227
  variation: hands behind back, 100, 101, 205, 209, 215, 227

Day-of-the-Week Practice
  Day 1, 200–201
  Day 2, 202–203
  Day 3, 204–205
  Day 4, 206–207
  Day 5, 208–209
  Day 6, 210–211
  Day 7, 212–213
Dhanurasana. See Bow Pose
Down-Plank Pose. *See* Up-Plank Pose and Down-Plank Pose (*Chaturanga Dandasana*)
Downward-Facing Dog Pose (*Adho Mukha Svanasana*)
  in back pain practice, 214
  in Busy Days Practice, 199
  in Day-of-Week Practice, 200, 203, 206, 208, 210, 212
  in fatigue practice, 229
  in flexibility practice, 217, 219
  overview, 67–71

in strength practice, 224
in 30 Poses Practice, 234
variation: Half-Dog at wall, 70,
    200, 214, 217, 219, 229
variation: toes on heel, 71, 206,
    208, 212

Elevated Legs-Up-the-Wall Pose
    (*Viparita Karani*)
in Busy Days Practice, 199
in Day-of-Week Practice, 201,
    203, 207, 212
in fatigue practice, 229
overview, 121–125
in relaxation practice, 231
in 30 Poses Practice, 234
variation: legs in bound angle
    pose, 123, 207, 229, 231
variation: legs in seated angle
    pose, 124, 203, 229, 231
Elliott, Theresa, 242
Encyclopedic Dictionary of Yoga, 2,
    196
energy, 226–228
Essential Breathing Practices
    (*Pranayama*), 191–193
#1: Even Inhalation, Even Exha-
    lation (*Sama Vrtti*), 192, 203,
    209, 213, 232
#2: Long Inhalation, Short
    Exhalation (*Visama Vrtti I*),
    192, 228
#3: Short Inhalation, Long
    Exhalation (*Visama Vrtti II*),
    193, 205, 211
in Day-of-Week Practice, 203,
    205, 209, 211, 213
in energy practice, 228
as limb of classical yoga, 2
recommendations, 191
in relaxation practice, 232
Even Inhalation, Even Exhalation
    (*Sama Vrtti*), 192, 203, 209, 213,
    232
Extended Side-Angle Stretch Pose
    (*Utthita Parsvakonasana*)
in Day-of-Week Practice, 204,
    208–209
in flexibility practice, 217
overview, 49–53
in strength practice, 224
in 30 Poses Practice, 233
variation: arm supported on
    thigh, 52, 53, 209
variation: hand on block, 52,
    204, 208, 217
Extended Triangle Pose (*Utthita
    Trikonasana*)

in balance practice, 222
in Busy Days Practice, 199
in Day-of-Week Practice, 200,
    202, 204, 206, 208, 210
in flexibility practice, 216
overview, 25–29
in strength practice, 224
in 30 Poses Practice, 233
variation: arm behind waist, 28,
    204, 206, 210, 222
variation: arm overhead, 28,
    208, 222
variation: facing wall, 28–29, 202
variation: hand on block, 27, 28,
    200, 216

fatigue, 229–230
Feuerstein, Georg, 2, 196, 241
flexibility practices, 216–218,
    219–221

glossary, 238–239
Goddesses in Everywoman, 7

Half-Dog Pose. *See* Downward-
    Facing Dog Pose (*Adho
    Mukha Svanasana*)
Half-Moon Pose (*Ardha Chan-
    drasana*)
in balance practice, 223
in Day-of-Week Practice, 202
in energy practice, 226
in flexibility practice, 216
overview, 31–35
in 30 Poses Practice, 233
variation: at wall with block, 34,
    35, 216
variation: hand on block, 34,
    202, 223
hamstring flexibility, 216–218
Head-of-the-Knee Pose (*Janu Sir-
    sasana*)
in Day-of-Week Practice, 203, 207
in flexibility practice, 217–218
overview, 145–149
in relaxation practice, 231–232
in 30 Poses Practice, 235
variation: foot back, 148, 149,
    207, 218, 232
variation: rolled blanket under
    bent knee, 148, 207, 217, 231
Headstand Preparation Pose
    (*Salamba Sirsasana*)
in balance practice, 223
in Day-of-Week Practice, 206,
    209
in flexibility practice, 220
overview, 85–89

in strength practice, 225
in 30 Poses Practice, 234
variation: feet on wall, 88, 209,
    220, 223, 225
variation: moving backward
    and forward, 87, 206, 220, 225
Hero-Heroine Pose (*Virasana*)
in Day-of-Week Practice, 203,
    213
in fatigue practice, 230
in flexibility practice, 220
overview, 139–143
in 30 Poses Practice, 235
variation: sitting on block, 142,
    203, 213, 230
variation: with arm stretch,
    142–143, 213
hip flexibility, 216–218
honoring oneself, 8, 198
humor, 9, 11

Iyengar, B. K. S. and Geeta, 2

Janu Sirsasana. See Head-of-the-
    Knee Pose
Jatara Parivartanasana. See Lying
    Twist Pose
joy of yoga, 4

Lasater, Judith, 196, 240, 243
Light on Yoga, 2
limbs of classical yoga, 2
Living Your Yoga, 196, 240
Long Inhalation, Short Exhala-
    tion (*Visama Vrtti I*), 192, 228
lower back pain, 214–215
Lunge Pose (*Anjaneyasana*)
in Day-of-Week Practice, 203,
    204, 210
in flexibility practice, 217
overview, 91–95
in 30 Poses Practice, 234
variation: back knee down, 93,
    204, 210, 217
variation: holding ankle, 94,
    203, 204, 210
Lying Twist Pose (*Jatara Parivar-
    tanasana*)
in back pain practice, 215
in Day-of-Week Practice, 201,
    205, 211, 213
in flexibility practice, 221
overview, 169–173
in 30 Poses Practice, 235
variation: feet wide apart, 171,
    201, 211, 215, 221
variation: on stack of blankets,
    172, 205, 213, 221

magazines, 241
Mantra Mats, 240
Mantras for Daily Practice
    Busy Days Practice, 199
    Day-of-Week Practice, 200, 202,
        204, 206, 208, 210, 212
    overview, 196
    Theme Practice, 214, 216, 219,
        222, 224, 226, 229, 231
    30 Poses Practice, 233
Miller, Barbara Stoller, 241
motivation, 8, 10, 11
Mountain Pose (*Tadasana*)
    in back pain practice, 214
    in balance practice, 222
    in Day-of-Week Practice, 200,
        202, 208
    overview, 15–17
    in 30 Poses Practice, 233
    variation: arms overhead, 17,
        200, 202, 208

niyamas (observances), 2, 6

Parsvottanasana. See Side-Chest
    Stretch Pose
Patanjali, 2
practice
    Busy Days Practice, 199
    Day-of-Week Practice, 200–213
    ending in Namaste, 196
    necessity for teachers, 10
    props for, 187, 197, 240
    sacred circle for, 7, 196
    sequencing, 196–197
    teaching as reflection of, 6
    Theme Practice, 214–232
    30 Poses Practice, 233–235
    tips, 197–198
pranayama. *See* Essential Breath-
    ing Practices
Prasarita Padottanasana. See
    Wide-Leg Standing Forward
    Bend Pose
props, 187, 197, 240
punctuality, 8, 10

Reclining Leg-Stretch Pose (*Supta
    Padangusthasana*)
    in back pain practice, 215
    in Day-of-Week Practice, 201,
        205, 207, 211
    overview, 163–167
    in 30 Poses Practice, 235
    variation: with strap, 166, 201,
        205, 207, 211, 215
Relax and Renew, 240
relaxation, 231–232

Relaxation (audio tape), 241
resources, 240–241
restraints (*yamas*), 2, 6
Rutter, Peter, 241

sacred circle, 7, 196
Salamba Sirsasana. See Headstand
    Preparation Pose
Sama Vrtti (Even Inhalation, Even
    Exhalation), 192, 203, 209, 213,
    232
Savasana. See Basic Relaxation
    Pose
Schatz, Mary Pullig, 241
Seated-Angle Pose (*Upavistha
    Konasana*)
    in Day-of-Week Practice, 203,
        207, 212
    in fatigue practice, 230
    in flexibility practice, 218
    overview, 151–155
    in relaxation practice, 232
    in 30 Poses Practice, 235
    variation: supported, 154, 155,
        212, 230, 232
    variation: with chair, 154, 207,
        218, 230, 232
sequencing
    Busy Days Practice, 199
    Day-of-Week Practice, 200–213
    overview, 196–197
    planning classes and, 3
    Theme Practice, 214–232
    30 Poses Practice, 233–235
Setu Bandhasana. See Bridge Pose
Sex in the Forbidden Zone, 241
Short Inhalation, Long Exhala-
    tion (*Visama Vrtti II*), 193, 205,
    211
shoulder flexibility, 219–221
Side-Chest Stretch Pose (*Parsvot-
    tanasana*)
    in Day-of-Week Practice, 206
    overview, 55–59
    in 30 Poses Practice, 233
    variation: halfway down, 58, 206
Simple Seated-Twist Pose
    (*Bharadvajasana*)
    in Busy Days Practice, 199
    in Day-of-Week Practice, 201,
        203, 205, 209
    in energy practice, 228
    overview, 133–137
    in 30 Poses Practice, 235
    variation: at wall, 136–137, 199,
        201, 228
socializing, 11
Standing Forward Bend Pose

    (*Uttanasana*)
    in Busy Days Practice, 199
    in Day-of-Week Practice, 201,
        207
    in energy practice, 226
    in fatigue practice, 230
    overview, 73–77
    in relaxation practice, 231
    in 30 Poses Practice, 234
    variation: hands on block, 75,
        201, 226, 230, 231
    variation: rolled mat under
        heels, 76, 207
    variation: rolled mat under toes,
        76, 77, 207
strength, 224–225
students. *See also* student-teacher
    relationship
    guidelines for class, 8–9
    relationship with oneself, 6
    responsibilities, 6, 7
    touching by teachers, 10–11
    transition to teacher, 9
student-teacher relationship
    boundaries, 6–7, 10–11, 12
    as mutual relationship, 3, 9
    school relationships versus, 6
    socializing, 11
    teacher's role, 7, 8
    touching, 10–11
Supported Shoulderstand Pose
    (*Salamba Sarvangasana*)
    in balance practice, 223
    in Day-of-Week Practice, 205,
        209, 211
    in energy practice, 228
    in flexibility practice, 221
    overview, 127–131
    in 30 Poses Practice, 234
    variation: balancing, 131, 223
    variation: one-legged, 130–131,
        223
    variation: with pole, 130, 221, 228
Supta Padangusthasana. See
    Reclining Leg-Stretch Pose

Tadasana. See Mountain Pose
teachers. *See also* student-teacher
    relationship
    burnout, 12
    code of ethics, 241
    criticizing other teachers, 11
    finding online, 241
    further study by, 12
    guidelines for, 9–10
    Lasater, 240, 243
    motivation, 10, 11
    practice and, 6

primary focus and adjustment, 3
questions to consider, 11–12
relationship with oneself, 6
self-interest in, 7
socializing with students, 12
student's transition to, 9
student's welfare and, 7
talking about other students, 11–12
touching by, 10–11
Theme Practice, 214–232
  for balance, 222–223
  for energy, 226–228
  in fatigue practice, 229–230
  for hip and hamstring flexibility, 216–218
  for lower back pain, 214–215
  for relaxation, 231–232
  for shoulder and upper back flexibility, 219–221
  for strength, 224–225
30 Essential Yoga Poses Practice, 233–235
time
  to hold poses, 198
  length of sessions, 198
  punctuality, 8, 10
touching, 10–11
Tree Pose (*Vrksasana*)
  in balance practice, 222
  in Day-of-Week Practice, 202, 204
  overview, 19–23
  in 30 Poses Practice, 233
  variation: hands at wall, 21
  variation: hands in Namaste, 22, 202, 204, 222
trust, 8, 10–11. *See also* boundaries

Upavistha Konasana. See Seated-Angle Pose
upper back flexibility, 219–221
Up-Plank Pose and Down-Plank Pose (*Chaturanga Dandasana*)
  in balance practice, 223

in Day-of-Week Practice, 203, 206, 209, 210
  in flexibility practice, 219
  overview, 79–83
  in strength practice, 224–225
  in 30 Poses Practice, 234
  variation: Up-Plank with hand up, 82, 209, 219, 223
Upward-Facing Bow Pose (*Urdhva Dhanurasana*)
  in Day-of-Week Practice, 205, 211
  in energy practice, 227–228
  in flexibility practice, 220–221
  overview, 115–119
  in 30 Poses Practice, 234
  variation: at wall with feet on blocks, 118, 119, 205, 211, 221, 228
  variation: at wall with hands on blocks, 117–118, 205, 211, 220, 227
Urdhva Dhanurasana. See Upward-Facing Bow Pose
Utthita Parsvakonasana. See Extended Side-Angle Stretch Pose
Utthita Trikonasana. See Extended Triangle Pose

Viparita Karani. See Elevated Legs-Up-the-Wall Pose
Virabhadrasana I. See Warrior I Pose
Virabhadrasana II. See Warrior II Pose
Virasana. See Hero-Heroine Pose
Visama Vrtti I (Long Inhalation, Short Exhalation), 192, 228
Visama Vrtti II (Short Inhalation, Long Exhalation), 193, 205, 211
Vrksasana. See Tree Pose

Warrior I Pose (*Virabhadrasana I*)
  in balance practice, 223

in Day-of-Week Practice, 200
  in energy practice, 226
  in flexibility practice, 216, 219
  overview, 37–41
  in strength practice, 224
  in 30 Poses Practice, 233
  variation: head back, 40, 219, 223
  variation: rolled mat under back foot, 39, 224, 226
Warrior II Pose (*Virabhadrasana II*)
  in Day-of-Week Practice, 200, 202, 206, 208, 210
  in energy practice, 226
  in flexibility practice, 216
  overview, 43–47
  in 30 Poses Practice, 233
  variation: back foot against wall, 46, 202, 216, 226
Web sites, 240, 241
Wide-Leg Standing Forward Bend Pose (*Prasarita Padottanasana*)
  in Day-of-Week Practice, 201, 204, 212
  in fatigue practice, 229
  in flexibility practice, 217
  overview, 61–65
  in 30 Poses Practice, 234
  variation: side twist, 64, 65, 212, 229
  variation: with block, 64, 201, 217, 229

yamas (restraints), 2, 6
yoga
  classical, 2
  joy of, 4
  resources, 240–241
Yoga: Discipline of Freedom, 241
Yoga Sutra of Patanjali, 2
Yoga Tradition, The, 241